Positive Medicine

Positive Medicine

Disrupting the Future of Medical Practice

DAVID BEAUMONT
MB ChB (Hons), MFOM, FAFOEM
Consultant Occupational Physician

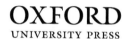

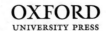

Great Clarendon Street, Oxford, OX2 6DP,
United Kingdom

Oxford University Press is a department of the University of Oxford.
It furthers the University's objective of excellence in research, scholarship,
and education by publishing worldwide. Oxford is a registered trade mark of
Oxford University Press in the UK and in certain other countries

First Edition published in 2021

Impression: 2

Published in the United States of America by Oxford University Press
198 Madison Avenue, New York, NY 10016, United States of America

British Library Cataloguing in Publication Data

Data available

Library of Congress Control Number: 2021936810

ISBN 978–0–19–284518–4

DOI: 10.1093/oso/9780192845184.001.0001

Printed and bound by
CPI Group (UK) Ltd, Croydon, CR0 4YY

Foreword

Positive Medicine travels along a narrow road that starts with a focus on illness and clinical interventions but leads to a wider highway where wellbeing and connectedness prevail. The journey traverses a tradition that religiously separated mind and body to a destination where mind and body become inextricably linked. Moreover, *Positive Medicine* affirms the wisdom of practising medicine in a setting where the patient is not separated from family or indeed from the social and cultural milieu that strengthens personal endurance.

In a system where human endeavours are fragmented into sectors and multiple disciplines, the essential nature of good health can be lost, and the brilliance of clinical wisdom can be lost to the less brilliant impacts from other external drivers that run counter to good health. Further, even when the most clearly visible determinants of health—determinants that can be quantified—are part of the medical purview, there is a dimension that lies beyond conventional quantification. It is apparent that the mind and the body are better understood now than they were four or five decades ago, and the significance of natural, social, and economic environments for health are increasingly part of an assessment and treatment process. But the profession has yet to embrace the relevance, and even the existence, of a spiritual dimension. For some, a spiritual experience may be part of a faith-based encounter; for others, it may be found within cultural traditions, or by the demonstration of compassion, or during encounters with the land, sea, or sky. For many indigenous cultures, that is not a new message. Improving health and wellbeing has always recognized the spirit as a motivating force for health.

Positive Medicine brings these multiple elements together and, in the process, lays foundations for a medical approach that goes beyond conventional practice. Strengthening the body, expanding the mind, fostering positive relationships, and lifting the spirit will challenge doctors to increase accustomed dimensions of practice. That will also require balancing medical science with other systems of knowledge such as indigenous knowledge—mātauranga Māori. It is never a question of one being 'right' and the other 'wrong'. Rather, it is about being ready to explore both and to know when one or the other will be better able to advance wellbeing.

Positive Medicine is a personal account of a journey that has inspired Dr Beaumont to go beyond the clinic and to enter the wider world of patients where mind, body, family, and spirit coexist. It is a journey that has relevance for all New Zealanders, if not for the wider world.

Titiro ki te pae tawhiti, te whitinga o te rā, te puāwaitanga o te mauri.
Look towards the distant horizon, the rising of the sun, and the flourishing of the people.

Mason Durie KNZM

Preface

When Ivan Illich published *Medical Nemesis* in 1974, he offered a withering critique of the medical profession and the medical model. 'The medical establishment has become a major threat to health.' Nearly half a century has elapsed since then, and things have got much worse.

In the healthcare systems of the UK, New Zealand, and Australia, a person might get an annual review with a doctor to check their blood pressure, blood sugar, and cholesterol, and perhaps obtain some lifestyle advice, but there is no time for any more. 'Health' in this context has a limited and very physical perspective. Having been a general practitioner (GP) in these systems, I understand the constraints of the 10-minute appointment.

In the UK, where healthcare is free at the point of contact, the system is so strained that the rule is often 'one problem per consultation'. Disease management takes precedence over disease prevention, and a wider perspective on health and wellbeing is largely absent.

In the UK, only 5 per cent of the health budget is spent on prevention.

But doctors want to practise differently. In 2019, the Royal College of General Practitioners conducted its largest-ever consultation of doctors and patients to develop a vision for the future of general practice. They learned that general practice is under 'huge strain', causing dissatisfaction among GPs and patients alike. GPs believe that the quality of patient care is suffering. At least once a month, one-third of GPs consider leaving the profession. Patients are being referred to secondary care simply because primary care cannot cope.

My aim in writing this book is to take up Illich's challenge, to understand the limitations of the medical model in which I was trained, and to propose a better approach. Back in the 1970s, Illich's book was seen as sensationalized and confrontational. It was the heyday of medical science. Medicine, and the power of doctors, were in the ascendant. But Illich's voice has finally been joined by others. One such is Seamus O'Mahony, the author of *Can Medicine be Cured?* (2019), a book that Richard Smith, a former editor of *The BMJ*, described as 'the most devastating critique of modern medicine since Ivan Illich'. Another is Sir Harry Burns, Professor of Global Health at Strathclyde University in Glasgow and former Chief Medical Officer for Scotland, who gave a talk to the Royal Australasian College of Physicians (RACP) Congress in 2016 called

'How doctors can change the world'. A third is Adam Kay in the book *This is Going to Hurt* (2017). His account of why he dropped out at the end of his specialist training in obstetrics and gynaecology to write for television is by turns funny and damning. And another is mine.

Unlike Illich, O'Mahony, and Kay, I believe medicine can be saved. In this book I explain how.

I term my alternative approach 'positive medicine'. I have reached this view after a long journey. I began working initially as a GP in the UK National Health Service, and I subsequently specialized as an occupational physician. I now practise in New Zealand. In various leadership roles within the RACP and my own faculty of occupational medicine, I have communicated aspects of this vision to my colleagues. Some have been resistant to the message that change is needed. But many have been open and receptive to what I have to say.

I now want to reach a broader audience of medical colleagues in the English-speaking world. There are many things about practising in New Zealand that have caused me to see things afresh, and I want to tell an international audience about them. One is the model of Māori health (te whare tapa whā—'four sides of the house of being') proposed by the distinguished psychiatrist and Māori scholar Sir Mason Durie. It fits well with the vision of empowerment proposed by Illich. Another is the insight I have gained as an occupational physician into the challenges of 'medically unexplained symptoms' and 'disability'.

The current healthcare system is a deficit model. It attempts to address and correct the absence of health, and is therefore more correctly termed a disease-care system. Positive medicine is an abundance model. It aims not only to help people manage illness and disease, but to enhance their health.

Although this book is very specifically about doctors and patients, it will resonate with all healthcare professionals. But as a doctor, my focus is on helping us get our own house in order.

Contents

Introduction

There Is a Third Way for Health

'Congratulations on a great Congress, David. But most of all, thank you, for permission to practise medicine how I've always known I should. I've wanted to work to a more holistic model, but I've been afraid of how my colleagues would react.'

The Royal Australasian College of Physicians (RACP) Congress 2019 in Auckland was the pinnacle of my professional career to date, and that moment made it all worthwhile. It was a milestone on my journey as a doctor. But it was much more than that.

The RACP is the professional body for all specialist physicians and paediatricians in New Zealand and Australia. Its Congress is the annual educational conference, for around one thousand doctors. I chaired the committee which put the programme together and invited experts in their field. We had disrupted the model, taken doctors to a new place in their learning. The theme was 'Impacting health along the life course'—the concept that our health is significantly influenced by our life journey, particularly from childhood, and that the keys to health lie in improving the ongoing life experience of our patients, and how we can influence that.

We had gone further, and identified that this is just as important for doctors themselves. Doctors are people too.

The gratitude of the specialist physician who felt he now had permission to practise medicine in a way that saw the patient as a whole person reflects a shift in the medical profession that I have been working towards for a long time. Two decades. It's my life's purpose. And it's not been easy.

Only last week I was talking to another doctor who practises 'whole-person medicine', a holistic model. He said, 'I've been doing this a long time now, David. It's been the toughest time of my life. When I started working this way, I got threats from my colleagues.'

I knew what he meant. I've had very lonely times, professionally, on my journey. I had only just started public speaking when I presented at a

Positive Medicine. David Beaumont, Oxford University Press. © Oxford University Press 2021.
DOI: 10.1093/oso/9780192845184.003.0001

prestigious New Zealand conference, the Goodfellow Symposium, in 2011. I was talking about the health benefits of work, presenting a review of the international evidence that work (specifically, *good* work) is beneficial to people's health.

I was halfway through my presentation when a hand shot up at the back. I hadn't anticipated questions at this stage, but maybe it would help clarify a point for the audience?

The doctor, a GP, said, 'Would you finish off the point you're making and summarize the rest of your talk? This is a complete waste of my time.'

Want to know what I did? I died on the stage. I finished off the point I was making, summarized the rest of my talk. Sat down. Broken.

I learnt so much from that experience. And I've never been fazed by it again. But it's an attitude that I've encountered time and time again. Only last year I was speaking at a medical conference about the need to explore the context of a person's life in understanding their symptom presentation. As I sat down, the chair, who was a GP, said to me, 'I'm going to use the chair's privilege to ask the first question.' It wasn't a question; it was a statement.

She said, 'If a patient comes in to see me to request an asthma inhaler, they don't want me to ask them what's happening in their lives!'

I pointed out the association between emotions and both production and severity of symptoms. But she wasn't having any of it. She persevered that it wasn't the role of a doctor to ask personal questions. 'And anyway, we don't have time.'

One of the doctors in the audience came up to me afterwards. With a grin on his face, he said, 'Great new way of thinking, David. I particularly enjoyed the fireworks afterwards!'

But this shouldn't be a new way of thinking. It is the reason I came into medicine, too many decades ago than I care to remember.

It's also *not* a new way of thinking to younger doctors and medical students. I've learned a lot about the way that medicine is now being taught from my son, Matt, who is now a junior doctor. Medical students are being taught about compassion and viewing the patient in the context of their whole lives, and concepts such as the 'biopsychosocial model', in ways that are not familiar to their senior doctors. (More on that later.)

Over the last 25 years I have been on a journey. Well, several journeys, actually. One is a journey to the realization that the medical model that doctors practise to, a model that has remained largely unchanged for 150 years, is no longer fit for purpose. Not on its own, in isolation. It needs more. The medical model is necessary but not sufficient. I've learnt that from the thousands of patients (clients) I have assessed who have been let down by the system. And by listening to doctors who are not practising medicine the way they want to. Because the healthcare system is not designed in that way.

Not least, *because there isn't enough time.*

Our healthcare systems are based on a deficit model. They aim to identify lack of health. And try to restore a degree of health. But they are failing even to do that, and losing the battle against many chronic diseases.

'Good news, the blood tests were all normal, the MRI scan was clear: you haven't got cancer!' That's the pinnacle of the medical model—congratulations, you've avoided a disease. That used to be good enough for patients, but not any more: 'So why have I got aches and pains all over? And why am I feeling tired all the time?'

There *is* an alternative. Many people, disgruntled with the traditional approach, are turning to a combination of personal development and alternative or complementary therapies. They are more likely to have someone spend time with them. And listen. The growth in the health and wellbeing sector in the last decade or so is testimony to what people are looking for. It has grown to an industry which is estimated to generate a global annual revenue of US$4.2 trillion. This has developed despite doctors and, other than the doctors working in integrated forms of practice, it largely exists *without* them.

Through the media of health and wellbeing books, online videos such as TED talks, Netflix documentaries, online personal development courses, and podcasts, people are developing health literacy. The Information Age means that information that used to be in the domain of doctors is now available to all. What used to be a power imbalance has shifted: 'I think I know more about my diabetes than my doctor does.' Not an uncommon refrain.

Another journey I've been on is my own personal journey from disease to health. To wholeness and healing. And it took more than physical treatment. This book tells that story too. I had to tell that story, because I have empathy for your stories. Because I have my own struggles too.

Who is this book written for? Doctors or patients?

I've been asked that question so many times, and my answer has always been the same. It's for people. Whether you're a doctor who feels you are not fulfilling your role to its full potential, or not prioritizing your own health. Whether you're a person who is fit and well, or not-so-fit and not-so-well, or whether you have developed overt disease, there are choices you can make.

This book intends to take you on the journey I have travelled, to help you reflect on your life and your health. Our way of life has led us to the level of health we have now. The choices we make now will impact our health into the future.

And the potential outcomes for those choices are massive. It's time to make positive choices.

For me, it led to a new and more satisfying model of practice: positive medicine.

Positive medicine takes the best of traditional medicine, adds the best of health and wellbeing practices, incorporates new sciences, and empowers people to develop positive health in every domain of our lives. In the process, it develops a new relationship between people and their doctors.

This book aims to overtly disrupt thinking and practice. This is a positive disruption. This is an innovative disruption. It methodically unpicks what isn't working and replaces it with something which intuitively is right. Fit for the future.

We must supplement the deficit model of medicine with an abundance model. Go beyond identifying and treating disease, beyond preventing disease, to enhancing health.

This is the third way. And it needs to be mainstream. It's about all of us.

1

Doctor Becomes Patient

The fourth of November 2003 is a day I will never forget. I was under pressure. A whole series of things, none amounting to anything dramatic on its own. But I was out of sorts, not feeling in control. In a word: *overwhelmed*.

I was driving home in heavy traffic. A miserable, wet, gloomy evening in northern England. A phone call from my wife, Susan: would I pick up some takeaway fish and chips on the way home? Make dinner easy. The kids were hungry.

The kids were aged 8 and 10 at the time. They were sat at the kitchen table, happy to see the dad they knew worked long hours. But I excused myself, said I needed to just sit in quiet for a few minutes before I could eat.

I didn't feel great. I was really tense. My chest was tight and it was an effort to breathe.

Susan came in to see if I was ready for dinner. She took one look at me and said, 'Shall I call a doctor?'

I said, 'Call an ambulance. Tell them I've got crushing central chest pain. Tell them I'm having a heart attack.'

I can picture vividly the journey in the back of the ambulance. 'Can you rate your pain on a scale of 1 to 10?'

It was 10. The injection that took the edge off the pain left me feeling spaced out. But I remember being shaken around as the ambulance went over speed bumps. They weren't hanging around and the sirens were going. I could see re-flections of the ambulance's blue lights in the buildings we went past.

In hospital, lots of people fussing over me. Another injection. Even more spaced out. I opened my dazed eyes to see my mother, grey with worry.

I don't remember the night at all. I remember waking early the next morning. The medical registrar pulled the curtains around my bed.

He said, 'Dr Beaumont, we've got most of your tests back and we think it's stress. It's not uncommon to feel the symptoms so intensely. We're still waiting for the results of your second cardiac enzymes, but assuming they're OK, you'll be able to go home. Why don't you take it easy for a couple of days?'

Positive Medicine. David Beaumont, Oxford University Press. © Oxford University Press 2021.
DOI: 10.1093/oso/9780192845184.003.0002

Intuitively, I knew he was wrong. An hour later the consultant cardiologist arrived with the ward sister (the senior nurse). He said, overly cheerily (I thought), 'Morning David, good to see you, sorry it's in these circumstances.'

I counted Richard as a friend. I was a local village GP, and he was the local cardiologist. We regularly met at hospital functions. I would often call him to discuss challenging patients. He sat on the edge of the bed and said, 'OK, we've had the final cardiac enzymes back. Significantly raised second enzymes. Combined with a good history and subtle ECG changes, you've had an NSTEMI.'

NSTEMI stands for 'non-ST elevation myocardial infarction'. It is a heart attack that does not extend through the full thickness of the heart muscle, but causes enough tissue damage to cause the cardiac muscles to release enzymes from dying cells, which proved it.

I'd had a small heart attack. At the age of 42. With no particular risk factors. Other than stress.

Richard performed an angiogram. It showed a narrowing in the coronary artery that had been occluded—blocked—with a blood clot which had now cleared. The narrowing didn't require any further intervention. No surgery was needed, and no stenting, which is when a small coil is inserted into the artery to widen the channel. I probably didn't need to be in hospital for nine days, but it was very reassuring to be there, nonetheless.

I was discharged from hospital on a cocktail of drugs aimed at reducing my risk of a further heart attack. I was given aspirin for blood thinning and to reduce platelet stickiness, a statin for cholesterol, and a beta-blocker to keep my blood pressure down and control my heart rate.

There was a twist to the story, as far as my relationship with the cardiologist was concerned. Richard was the first doctor I'd ever treated as a patient.

I was a young, newly qualified doctor, having gone straight into general practice from my junior doctor hospital rotations. I saw his name on my list of patients for that morning. Here was me as a new GP, seeing a consultant cardiologist for a health problem! I was very nervous as he walked into the room. After exchanging pleasantries, he said, 'Would you have a look at this pigmented lesion on my back?' I relaxed a little, my confidence growing. I'd just finished a dermatology job as part of my hospital rotations. There, in the centre of his back, was a black, warty-looking skin lesion, about 2 cm across.

I was probably too blasé, but with the confidence of certainty I said, 'Oh, that's a seborrheic keratosis. Nothing to worry about, benign and very common as the skin starts to age. They actually scrape off the surface very easily with a curette, and we can send it off for histology.'

It might have felt straightforward to me, but I saw a look of relief on his face and saw his shoulders relax. Suddenly I realized what, on reflection, should have been obvious. Richard had come to see me because he was worried that it might be a malignant melanoma. The worst kind of skin cancer. Why wouldn't he? They actually look very similar unless you've seen lots.

My biggest realization was that he wasn't just a consultant cardiologist, he was also a patient. In fact, he had come to me as a patient and deserved (and expected) to be treated as such. Doctors with medical concerns, just like any patient with medical concerns, come to a doctor in a state of apprehension at least, and often fear about what the outcome may be.

That was my very first realization that doctors are patients too.

From that time, I never had any problem treating doctors, and in fact have seen many professionally for their own health over the course of my career. But it's not always like that. Research shows that doctors are not good at looking after their own health and don't seek medical attention when they should. Often, they don't even have their own GP (and therefore may treat themselves). When they do seek help from another doctor, they often receive substandard care, specifically because they are not treated like a patient. The assumption is made that they understand the medical terminology, so normal explanations and reassurance are not required. Hospital 'corridor consultations' are common.

But here I was, discharged from hospital after a small heart attack. It was my turn to be doctor-as-patient. I was a good patient; I did as I was instructed and took the tablets meticulously. Still do—they are my friends; they are reducing my risk factors for further heart problems.

I made some lifestyle changes. On reflection, probably not enough (and not sustained). I started walking on a daily basis, albeit slowly. I started doing more about the house, including mowing the lawns. I recall the startling realization about how much the heart attack had changed me when one day, as I came back into the house, Susan said, 'I just watched you mowing the lawns. I'm concerned. You looked like an old man.'

I certainly felt changed. More vulnerable; perhaps even fragile.

However, at 4 weeks post heart attack I went for my out-patient review. I had a stress ECG (monitoring of the heart electrical activity while under the strain of walking at increasing speed and elevation on a treadmill). It was perfect. So was my blood pressure and cholesterol. Everything was back to normal, and I was discharged.

It was at this point that my senior doctor said to me, 'We're really pleased at the progress you're making with your recovery, but we're worried about your state of mind. We'd like you to see a psychologist.'

It was the sort of advice that I might have given, so I agreed, and had six sessions with an amazing psychologist called Bryce. He specialized in middle-aged men, and my situation was not unfamiliar to him. I told him that I had been on a career progression, that my life was unfolding before me, but now I'd had a heart attack. It had all gone.

He challenged me, 'What if I said to you that nothing has changed? What if you can get back on the trajectory? What if your heart attack doesn't matter?'

This was not the way I saw it initially, but gradually I came round to thinking that I couldn't fault his logic. There was more to my health than just physical recovery from the heart attack.

Leaving general practice

By the time of my heart attack, I had left general practice to become a specialist doctor in the field of occupational medicine. I had become a quite rare breed of doctor (which many people haven't even heard of) called an occupational physician. I had specialized in the health of workers.

The move was all thanks to the senior partner in the general practice I had joined after leaving hospital medicine. Not long after I had joined the practice, he came into my consultation room and said, 'David, there's a transport company down the road that is looking for a company doctor. That's something you would be interested in.'

It wasn't a question, it was a statement, and as a dutiful junior partner I took up the new role.

I found I enjoyed the interaction with the workers, many of whom were seasoned truck drivers and very down to earth and blunt. Although they treated me with some respect, there was a certain flippancy and cheekiness about the way they greeted me.

'Morning, Doc. What are you up to today?'

For me, there was something reassuring about being treated like one of the team, because I felt I was. I was looking after the guys so they could do their job. I had a part to play. Any respect had to be earned and not be given just because of my title. This was further emphasized by the fact that they didn't come to me at the surgery. I had to go to them, at the transport base. I examined them in the tiny first aid room. I ate with them in their canteen. I heard the stories of the things that were happening in their lives; the things that mattered to them.

One thing that didn't matter to them as much as it should have was their health. Most of them were in the dangerous demographic of being middle-aged men. At 42, I had been young to have a heart attack and had no specific risk factors. But they were in their 50s and 60s—overweight, hypertensive, smokers with elevated cholesterol, doing sedentary work as drivers. Even worse, this demographic has very poor health-seeking behaviour. They don't like going to see doctors, and are often poorly compliant with medical advice. So, I did their health checks at work, and told them what measures they should take to improve their health. Yes, I told them what to do, not that most of them paid a blind bit of notice.

Well, not until one of them dropped dead from a massive heart attack the day after I had done a routine medical.

As I reviewed his file, I decided that there was nothing I could have done to prevent his heart attack. In fact, of all the team, his risk profile for cardiac events was lower than most. Part of my job was to identify that people were fit to do their job and, specifically, met the legislative requirements to be considered fit to drive a heavy vehicle. I had found nothing the previous day to suggest I should have stopped him driving. Thankfully for other road users, his heart attack had not occurred while he was behind the wheel of his truck. It did, however, make his mates more attentive when I did their medicals.

The senior partner in the practice who had convinced me to be a company doctor subsequently came to me and said, 'Competence issues in medicine are becoming increasingly important in medical practice. You need a postgraduate qualification to support your company doctor work. We'll fund you to do the new Diploma in Occupational Medicine.'

This proved to be a wise suggestion. It anticipated the increasing accountability for competence that doctors need to have.

I subsequently gained higher qualifications, and started doing less time in general practice and more in various workplaces. Increasingly, I become conscious of the differing roles I had in people's lives in the workplace compared with in the consultation room. One of the key differences was the degree of formality and level of relationship.

In the surgery, I was only ever known as 'Dr Beaumont'. Respect came from the title. In the workplace, though, I was more likely to be called 'Doc'. My role was different too. It was far more about keeping people healthy, or helping them get back to work after an illness or injury, or advising employers about making adjustments at work so that people with a disability could be helped to stay in work. My work was becoming to be about health and prevention, and not about disease and treatment.

This became the case to such an extent that I didn't prescribe in my at-work role. That was left to people's own GPs. In fact, because I did not hold responsibility for the medical treatment of the people I saw at work, they were officially not my patients. I therefore referred to them as clients—and still do.

Inevitably, I left general practice to specialize in the evolving and exciting field of occupational medicine.

Before long, I was working in a fantastic role that had me visiting mines and quarries, chemical plants, heavy engineering works, food manufacturers, even hospitals, where I looked after the health of the doctors, nurses, and ancillary staff. In fact, somehow *The BMJ* got hold of the story of my new-found career and contacted me to ask if I would write a piece to include in the Career Focus section .

The piece appeared, illustrated by a photo of me, grinning like a Cheshire cat, with the chimneys, pipework, and tanks of a chemical plant in the background under the headline, 'My dream job'. Years later, a young occupational physician came up to me at a conference and told me that reading my article had inspired her to leave general practice too, to follow the same specialty.

There was another event that led me to question further my relationship with patients.

Not long after the heart attack, I saw a client called John for a travel medical at his place of work. He had also been a patient of mine when I had been a GP. John was a big guy, in every sense of the word. He was tall, overweight, and had a big personality. He drank and smoked too much and had a very high-pressure job. Every time I saw him, I would tell him he was a 'ticking time-bomb', and that his heart attack was only a matter of time.

On this occasion, it became evident to me very quickly as he came into the room that he had heard that I had suffered a heart attack. With glee he said, 'Isn't it ironic that for all that time you told me I had to change my lifestyle, and you're the one who had the heart attack!'

I'm sure I smiled sweetly at him, but under my breath I muttered a few choice words.

Over the years, I've reflected on my approach to health promotion with my patients, and realize that it amounted to paternalism. I'll explain what that means, but first, here is the parody of the consultations I used to have with John: 'Lose some weight, stop smoking, cut down your alcohol, get a better work–life balance. Come back in a month's time and I'll recheck your blood pressure.'

In fairness, it was as much of a system failure as it was my fault. At least the advice was given in addition to prescribing medication. My training in what to say and how to say it had been sketchy at best. On the other hand, I had only 7½ minutes to spend with him (because in UK general practice we had eight appointments per hour). That is not nearly enough time to deal with the presenting problem and hope to positively influence his lifestyle.

Paternalism and patients

The concept of paternalism in the doctor–patient relationship suggests that it is inherently hierarchical. There is a power imbalance based on a knowledge imbalance: the doctor knows what's best for you and therefore can tell you what to do. The implication is that you should comply.

At best, this approach must be considered condescending and demeaning, but at its worst, it is disingenuous.

It is worth capturing this description of the 'paternalistic doctor' by a UK GP from 1992 (back when I was in general practice), Dr Brian McInstry:

> In this relationship, the general practitioner listens to the patient, believing that a doctor who listens is a more effective doctor. The general practitioner genuinely wants the best for the patient but believes that patients often need to be guided firmly through the decision-making process as they do not always know what is best for them. The general practitioner is prepared to answer questions about the illness and will even acquiesce with certain less important suggestions. For example, a general practitioner treating a patient with hypertension would be willing to make several changes in therapy for the patient. However, if the patient suggested stopping the treatment, the general practitioner would feel justified in exaggerating the possible unpleasant sequelae of this action, citing for example that 'you would almost certainly have a stroke'. Even though the general practitioner knows this to be untrue. This is justified in the doctor's mind as he or she considers that the long-term interests of the patient would be better served by the patient having the treatment despite its unpleasant side effects, regarded as minor by the doctor.[1]

I sincerely hope I was not guilty of deliberately exaggerating to John. I don't believe so. But nevertheless, the conversation with John has led me to consider more deeply the doctor–patient relationship, and what each expects from the other. In particular, what is the form of this relationship that best serves the patient? What best serves both parties, patient and doctor?

Even the word 'patient' has been criticized as reinforcing the imbalance between the carer and the recipient of health services. Julia Neuberger, formerly Chair of the UK Patients' Association, has argued for doing away with the word altogether. She pointed out that the word comes from the Latin word *patiens*, which means 'one who suffers':

> The word 'patient' conjures up a vision of quiet suffering, of someone lying patiently in a bed waiting for the doctor to come by and give of his or her skill, and of an unequal relationship between the user of healthcare services and the provider ... The patient, in this language, is truly passive—bearing whatever suffering is necessary and tolerating patiently the interventions of an outside expert ... The healthcare professional is the healer, while the recipient is the healed, and does not need to take part in any decision making or in any thinking about alternatives.[2]

If the paternalistic doctor sounds patronizing, Dr Brian McKinstry also described the type of doctor he called the 'autocratic doctor':

> The doctor has little regard for the opinions of the patient. The patient has come to consult the expert with a problem ... Questions from the patient about the treatment are considered irritating as they signify a lack of recognition of the general practitioner's abilities, or a sign of ignorance on the part of the patient ... The doctor believes that the patient is lucky to have the benefit of expert advice and the patient is being ungrateful if it is not accepted. For such doctors, patients exist for the sake of medicine rather than medicine existing for the sake of patients.[3]

I'm cringing as I type the words, yet I know I have met doctors of both the paternalistic and the autocratic types.

I now don't use the word 'patient' to describe the people I see. When I'm talking to them, I use their first name, and ask them to call me by mine. When I'm talking about them, I use the word 'client'. However, since the purpose of this book is to describe the failings of the current system and to present a way forward to a new relationship, I will continue to use the conventional word patient until that new model is fully revealed.

Doctors are people too

I had another 'doctor becomes patient' moment shortly before I left general practice; one that stretched my understanding of the doctor–patient relationship still further.

It started with a pink eye. Sore and watering. It became painful and was associated with blurred vision in my right eye. Clearly, you shouldn't take risks with eyes but, being a doctor, I couldn't resist doing the first check myself.

I did what I would have done for a patient and got some fluorescein from the fridge. Fluorescein is a yellow dye that fluoresces under ultraviolet (UV) light. The practice had a blue UV light specially for the purpose, and I turned the lights down in my consultation room and looked in the mirror. Sure enough, I saw what I was expecting. I had a corneal ulcer, a small hole in the cornea that covers the iris (the coloured part of the eye whose hole forms the pupil).

It was worse than that, as the hole was over the top part of the pupil, which is why it was affecting my vision. Worse still, the bright yellow fluorescence that stained the hole (as it was glowing in the UV light) had small, spidery legs running from its centre in all directions. These are called dendrites (which simply means 'tree-like shapes'). I had a dendritic corneal ulcer, which is typically caused by the herpes virus.

I got an appointment for the hospital eye clinic the same day and my self-diagnosis was confirmed. I was started on an antiviral eye ointment. Surprisingly, about an hour after applying the ointment (four times a day), it made me feel dreadful. Hard to describe, but a sort of cross between headache and nausea.

The next morning, I was truly struggling to get through morning surgery. Two and a half hours, and 20 patients to see.

The last patient came into the room: Eileen, a 74-year-old woman. She said, 'I've just come back from the funeral. My son had a massive heart attack. No mother should have to bury her son.'

I took a deep breath to start to address her grief. As soon as I did, I felt a lump welling in my throat. I felt myself tearing up. I reached across the desk to take her hand, thinking that if I touched her hand it would spur me on to offer my condolences, but of course it only made my emotions keener. My sadness was absolutely for the raw humanness of her situation, but it was also for myself, and the realization that I really wasn't coping. (In truth, I shouldn't have been at work at all.)

We sat in silence for what must have been 15 minutes, my hand touching hers. She sat with her head bowed. Tears silently flowing down her cheeks. She got up. Left the room. Neither of us said a word. Not even goodbye.

After that, I didn't go back to work for a week, until the corneal ulcer had healed. For a long time, I believed I had let Eileen down that day, that I hadn't fulfilled my role as a doctor. Hadn't reached for the prescription pad.

Then it hit me. I may not have fulfilled my role as a doctor (in fact, I was not fit to be in the role of doctor that day), but I did fulfil the role of a human being. Of all that I could have done, probably the best thing was to give her human touch and a silent acknowledgement of her pain and grief. It is only recently that I have learnt this action has a term; it is called 'holding space'.

I would like to believe that she walked out in silence that day, not because she felt that it was a waste of my time, but because she had felt heard in the most innately human way.

And it helped me to realize that doctors are people too.

Where to from here?

You've met me now.

I suspect you know more about me and my life than you do about your own doctor. I have been a very traditional doctor, and my medical school training was very traditional. My current medical practice is mainstream, but I would not describe it as traditional. I will describe the way I practise in detail.

This book is written for both patients and doctors, and indeed also for doctors taking the role of patient, as I have experienced. I will share more of my personal story, which I regard as providing important context for you to realize that I understand the pain that everyone goes through as patients. And, of course, we are all patients at various points in our lives.

My understanding of what patients need from doctors and from healthcare came first from my own experience as a patient. And, of course, our experience of health and illness occurs against the backdrop of the experience of life events. I can speak from that perspective too, I've had plenty of life experiences, which gives me the ability to empathize about your circumstances too.

Some years ago, while formulating my concepts around the relationship between doctors and patients, I googled the phrase 'doctors are people too'. I found very few references to this then-radical concept. Two that I did find were these: first, a journalistic article by a guy who went to see his doctor and used the throwaway question, 'And how are you today, doctor?' He was very surprised to be told that the doctor was having a tough time at the moment because there was a lot going on in his life. This caused him to stop and reflect: 'That's when I realized that doctors are people too.'

The second reference was to an amazing doctor called Sam Hazledine, who has devoted his career to helping improve the lives of doctors, by improving their working circumstances and helping them focus on their own health and wellbeing. I have come to know Sam well, and I will talk more about how his work has impacted the role of doctors as people and the health of doctors in a later chapter.

Googling the phrase 'doctors are people too' today, I find there are many, many more references to this concept. Most are written by doctors, and these are a plea by doctors for patients and the system to recognize that doctors are only human.

Society has come to expect too much of doctors, imbuing them with almost superhuman powers. That's a very tough act to live up to, and one that can only go wrong. There is a whole science of understanding the mistakes doctors make. And estimates of rates of incorrect diagnosis vary between 10 and 20 per cent. If doctors are people too, then to err is human.

Societal expectations on doctors also limit personal responsibility. Expectations that a doctor will identify a diagnosis and provide treatment are so strong that it creates a sense of going to see a doctor to be fixed, much as we take our car to the garage to get fixed. This book will identify clearly that the human body doesn't work like that. Rather, the answers lie in us taking control of our own health.

Many of the pleas for understanding of the humanness of doctors come from younger doctors, especially junior doctors in their quest for better working hours and conditions. These are the words of Dr Michelle Au:

> We want our doctors to be perfect. We want them to know all the answers, to never say the wrong thing, and above all, to always, always, be there for us. We want our doctors to be superhuman. But the fact of it is: *they're not.* Doctors are not perfect, they're not beyond mortal concerns. After working 30 hours straight, they get tired, and that interferes with their ability to work well. After being in the hospital for three weeks without a single day off, they get burned out. When they get sick, sometimes it's hard for them to come to work (though, to be honest, we are terrible hypocrites and most of us come in anyway). They are young adults, and sometimes, they want to have connections outside of work—friends, spouses, children, and a reasonable amount of time to spend with them. These are not ridiculous things to ask for. These are not unthinkable standards to expect.[4]

My own learning was that there is more to health than physical recovery. I also learnt that doctors are people too, and some doctors at least want this to be recognized.

So, what do patients want?

The European Patients' Forum has articulated this clearly. They say they want empowerment. 'Patient empowerment is a process that helps people gain control of their own lives and increase their capacity to act on issues that they themselves define as important.'[5] They say that empowerment includes confidence and coping skills to be able to manage their own health and conditions, including education and developing expertise in these areas. They want to develop self-awareness and self-efficacy—a belief that they have the ability to take control of their own life and health.

To do this, they ask for equality: 'Patients need support to become equal partners with health professionals in the management of their conditions.'[6]

Now we're starting to see that, rather than the old-school, traditional, hierarchical, doctor–patient relationship, we have the makings of a doctor–patient *partnership*. (Or better still, a doctor–person partnership.) This is the basis for patient-centred care, perhaps better known as person-centred care.

What we need to deliver this interaction is both a new model of practice for doctors, and a shared understanding between doctors and people that the old paradigm has been superseded by a new way of defining the relationship. This changes the respective roles, empowering people without detracting from the need for expertise from the doctors, and in return giving people more responsibility for their own health.

My personal experience of working to this new model is that it increases satisfaction for both the doctor and the person being cared for.

2

There's Something Wrong

As an occupational physician, one of my main roles is to help people return to work after an illness or injury, usually referred by an employer and an insurer or a workers' injury compensation body. In New Zealand, this body is called the Accident Compensation Corporation (ACC). In my years in practice in New Zealand, and prior to that in the UK, I have seen and assessed thousands of people who have not gone back to work when it would have been expected that they would. Many of these people have been let down by the system, including by their doctors.

The system fails people

As an expert in what goes wrong, I have become increasingly aware of what success might look like. As I have understood more about why things go wrong and harm people's health, I have realized that system changes, and changes to medical provision in particular, could not only prevent ill health and disability but *improve* people's health.

To bring about these changes, two things need to happen: first, people need to realize there is a problem; and second, the will to change has to be strong enough to change the way things have been done for decades, even centuries. And the reward must be big enough for the effort required. I believe these parameters can easily be met, for individuals, families, and communities. The changes to healthcare systems that can occur would bring massive economic benefits.

The seminal day in my professional career came early in my work as a specialist in the health of workers, around 2002. I received a referral from an employer to see a 30-year-old factory worker who had injured his shoulder. He had received physiotherapy and was on the mend, but his return to work was delayed. I met with Joe at his place of work and, together with his health and safety manager, we went to have a look at his job on the factory floor. Joe

Positive Medicine. David Beaumont, Oxford University Press. © Oxford University Press 2021.
DOI: 10.1093/oso/9780192845184.003.0003

and his colleagues demonstrated what was involved in his work tasks and we agreed that his shoulder limitations (inability to elevate his arm above shoulder height) meant that there were aspects of the job he was unable to do. However, there were also clearly parts of his job that he *could* usefully do. Together we devised and agreed a return-to-work programme with gradually increasing hours and gradually increasing duties.

Since he was off work with a sick note (a medical certificate issued by his GP), I wrote to his GP describing the programme and asking that he sign him off to return to work on the following Monday. I received a quick response from his GP, with a brief letter that stated: 'This is my patient. I decide when he's fit for work.'

I was astounded. Although I was still new to rehabilitation for work, I was a specialist in this area. I thought I was meant to be the 'expert'. With no clue as to what to do, I contacted the health and safety manager and asked him what would happen next.

He said, 'Nothing. There's nothing we can do. He's got a sick note; he can't come back to work.' And he didn't.

Honestly, I was reeling. It just felt so wrong. He was a young guy who was being prevented from getting back to work, and getting on with his life. From an employment perspective, it had very serious ramifications. From my own professional point of view, I was left asking: so, what value do I add anyway?

At the time, I was just getting into medical politics: the concept that doctors have positions of influence that can be used to advocate for positive change. I was on the Council of the Society of Occupational Medicine (SOM) in London. I took my problem to the next Council meeting, excited for my senior colleagues to enlighten me as to what I could have done. What I heard shocked me even more. Around the table, doctor after doctor said, 'Oh yes, happens all the time. It's just one of those things. GPs don't get the relationship between health and work.'

So, on to the next item of business for the SOM Council meeting.

But then the president, Dr John Challenor, said, 'Look, this is clearly a big problem, but it's really hard to know what to do about it. It would take a complete change in behaviour. David, why don't you contact the Royal College of General Practitioners [RCGP] and just test out whether they see it as a problem?'

So, I phoned the chair of Council for the RCGP (London), Dr David Haslam. Again, I was filled with trepidation. Here was I, a new specialist in occupational medicine, questioning the most senior professional GP in the country about why GPs were causing a problem. He was fantastic (phew!). He told me that, unfortunately, the situation I described with Joe was not uncommon, and that the role of GPs in rehabilitation and return to work was fraught with problems. For a start, most GPs had no training in this area. They didn't have the time in a consultation to go through the assessment of fitness for work, and often the easiest thing to do was simply to write a sick note. He also said that GPs didn't want to fall out with their patients, or to damage the doctor–patient relationship. In fact, he told me, many GPs considered that it shouldn't be their role in the first place. He suggested a couple of people I could talk to, to understand more of what was happening.

As I spoke to more and more people in very influential positions, I began to realize the scale of the problem. This was massive. It was a system failure of epic proportions. I decided that it needed researching and publishing.

Anyone who has ever done any form of research will know that the first job is to decide what we already know about a subject. So, I undertook a literature review of the world research into the role of GPs in rehabilitation and return to work. It didn't take me long, because there was next to nothing out there. There were a few papers from the Netherlands where, by law, anyone off work for a certain period of time had to be seen and assessed by an occupational physician. What the research papers were saying was that this created significant tension and conflict between the GPs who were signing people off work and the occupational physicians who were trying to help them get back to work. (As ridiculous as that sounds to me as I type it.)

I found one reference from the UK written by a fellow occupational physician, Dr John Gration. He had written an opinion piece in the *Journal of Occupational Medicine*. The very opening paragraph read:

'We obviously have conflicting interests. Mine is the well-being of my patient and yours is returning him to productive work.' Such comments may be thought attributable to a nineteenth-century reformer in communication with a despotic mine owner, in fact they were not, but were received by me from a GP after I had written to him concerning a patient whose extended sickness absence was due to anxiety and depression.[1]

This captured everything! We occupational physicians were trying to help people get back to work, and the GPs (these particular GPs) were actively working against this. There was a perceived conflict of interest, with the welfare of the patient right at the centre of the disagreement, based on two very different models of belief about the role of work in people's lives. When I did publish my research, and presented it in London at the Annual Scientific Meeting of the SOM, a former president of the Society, Dr Roy Archibald, who must have been well into his 80s at the time, stood up and said, 'It's been this way for as long as I can remember.'

When little is already known about a subject, it makes the subject difficult to research. Where do you start? Thankfully, I found a research methodology called a Delphi study. In Ancient Greece, if you wanted to answer to a difficult question you went to the source of wisdom, the Oracle at Delphi. In this method, a group of expert informants are approached and asked for their opinion. The researcher (me) documents the opinions and searches for common themes. These are collated and fed back to the experts, who comment as to whether the themes and concepts are correct. There are three rounds of going backwards and forwards (iterations) until a statement has been produced that all experts are agreed upon.[2]

I spoke to very senior GPs, occupational physicians, nurses, and physiotherapists, but also employers' representatives, union representatives (the Trades Union Congress, or TUC), and the government (the Department for Work and Pensions). They made my job very easy, because they all said the same kind of things. They identified the problem and causes and came up with some solutions. They readily agreed to put their names to the statement, which was then published (the consensus statement is in Appendix 2),[3] which prompted an editorial in *The BMJ*.[4] This highlighted the downsides of the effects of poor communication between the two groups, GPs and occupational physicians, together with the evidence that GPs who participate in minimizing their patients' disability achieve better health outcomes as well as greater patient satisfaction.

A key extract from the consensus statement is that:

GPs play a crucial role in work absence because they see many patients with chronic illness and disability, they co-ordinate and provide effective clinical management and they provide sick notes which trigger or continue periods of absence from work.

Some GPs are not aware how influential their role is, or the beneficial effect that work can have on their patients' health.

That was it. That was why the problem had arisen to block Joe's return to work. His GP had no realization as to the importance of helping Joe get back to work, and had actively blocked it, with the potential for him to lose his job. The GP did not realize how important work was to Joe and his family.

From that time there has been a considerable amount of research into this problem. One of the methods which has been very effective in unpicking the problem is focus groups. Groups of GPs are invited by the researchers to participate in a discussion about the topic. Their answers are captured and the themes are collated. One of the most prolific investigators in this field is Professor Debbie Cohen, herself a former GP. Together with Professor Sir Mansel Aylward, she led a team of researchers asking GPs about their attitudes to patients being out of work long term and referring them to rehabilitation services.

Their published paper and the collected comments from the GPs make fascinating reading. You can almost hear the puzzlement in the GPs' voices as to why they are being asked about this topic, because it's not a medical question:

> Obviously my role isn't that [*seeing patients for being out of work*] unless they have an illness for which they need medical help … but if it's just purely because they're out of work I don't personally think that's a GP role.

And:

> We don't see that [*referring patients for rehabilitation*] as our primary role … our role is health … and primary health and prevention.

The conclusions they reached from the study were that:

> There was consensus among participants that the management of long-term worklessness was not part of the GP's role. Participants described clearly their feelings about the boundaries that existed between managing their patients' health and managing long-term worklessness.

And:

> GPs did not feel that discussion about work-related issues with their patients was of high importance nor part of their role and as a consequence did not routinely enquire about work or attitudes about returning to employment.[5]

One of my own experiences of exactly this perspective was when I called a GP to let him know that an insurance company was funding me to provide a rehabilitation programme to help his patient get back to work after 3 years off work with chronic fatigue syndrome. (The patient had an income protection policy which provided a rehabilitation benefit.)

He said, 'Well they would, wouldn't they? They just want to get him off claim.' I pointed out that if he came off his income protection claim, that meant that he had returned to work sustainably, which was surely the best thing for him? But the GP was clearly unconvinced.

On another occasion I was seeing John, who had also been off work for 3 years following a back injury. A magnetic resonance imaging (MRI) scan had shown an annular tear of one of the discs in his lumbar spine. In truth, such a tear is a common occurrence and a common finding in the general population. He sat down in my office. I commenced with an introduction and explanation of my role in providing assessment and advice regarding his rehabilitation and return to work. I felt it coming before it happened. He was sat with his arms folded, eyes rolling, huffing and puffing.

He reached into his pocket and banged a piece of paper down on the desk, hard. 'That's for you!'

It was a letter from his GP. It was indeed addressed to me. I still have that letter, I was so shocked by it. It said:

Dear Dr Beaumont,

I have been very clear previously that all attempts to get John back to work should cease. It is ridiculous that he should have to go through this process when he obviously would be better remaining off work. He should remain a long-term beneficiary. He is taking legal advice and I will be supporting him.

I calmly said to John, 'How do you feel, that your GP is suggesting that all attempts to help you should cease and that you should remain a disabled person?'

He looked puzzled and said, 'He's not saying that . . .'

I replied, 'That's exactly what he is saying.'

At this point his partner stepped in. (John was 38 and had a partner and three children.)

She said, angrily, 'Well, it's not what we want! We don't want him lying on the couch watching TV all day and being grumpy with us. We want him back at work!'

Suitably chastised, John turned to me and said, 'Well, of course, there's nothing I want more than to get back to work. The last time they tried to get me back they had me as a caretaker. I had to ride a mower across bumpy ground and it just made me worse.'

The impasse had been broken.

I was able to agree with him and say that was not an appropriate duty for someone with back problems, at least in the early stages of recovery. The assessment (which would take an hour, and look at all aspects of John and his life) then proceeded in a far more positive manner, and we agreed a way forward. John had a multidisciplinary rehabilitation programme, with a physiotherapist, occupational therapist, and psychologist (to help him with his understanding of pain, and the value to him and his family of recovery of function to get on with his life). Three months later, he was on a return-to-work programme and successfully got a job.

I should say at this point that New Zealand is fortunate to have what is probably the best injury compensation scheme in the world: ACC. It is based on the principle of 'no fault', so to be able to receive treatment, rehabilitation, and even weekly wage compensation does not depend on having to sue somebody for the injury.

Time to join a committee and make a difference

After my heart attack and the family move to New Zealand, I took a break from medical politics. We had been in New Zealand for about 3 years, when my wife said to me, 'David, it's not like you not to be on a committee!'

The professional body for all specialist occupational physicians in New Zealand and Australia is the Australasian Faculty of Occupational and Environmental Medicine (AFOEM), which is part of the Royal Australasian College of Physicians (RACP). I went to their Annual Scientific Meeting for the first time in 2009. I was on a mission: to find Dr Mary Wyatt. I had been told that she was the chair of the AFOEM's Policy and Advocacy Committee, which was the route for me to get on a committee that made a difference.

At lunch time on the first day of the conference, I asked a colleague if he knew who Mary Wyatt was. Without hesitation, he said, 'That's her!' I immediately shot after her. She said, 'Haven't got time to talk. Just going to a committee meeting; why don't you come with me?'

So, I got into my first Policy and Advocacy Committee meeting by accident (I'm a firm believer in *meant to be*). A new project was presented at the meeting, called 'The adverse health consequences of long-term worklessness'. It was clear that international evidence was demonstrating that being out of work long term was harmful to health, and that solutions were required. They needed someone to lead the team investigating and developing the project. An ideal opportunity for me to volunteer and get the job!

I pointed out that the evidence was clear that being out of work was harmful to health but, increasingly, evidence was coming out of the UK that the corollary was also true: that something about work itself was good for health. We agreed that a positive slant would be good, and the title of the project became 'Realising the Health Benefits of Work'. There was a play on words: 'realising' meaning to become aware of or recognize or make clear; and 'realising' meaning to make real, make happen.

We launched the position statement, *Realising the Health Benefits of Work*, in 2010.[6] Professor Sir Mansel Aylward agreed to do the launch presentation for us, coming out from the UK and launching it in both New Zealand and Australia. It was a true trans-Tasman project. At the launch were senior representatives from many different medical and allied healthcare professions, and also representatives of the government, employers, and unions. It was clear that the implications for the concept that work was good for health had ramifications for many different stakeholders. I chaired the launch, and pointed out that there seemed to be agreement that we all had a vested interested in getting this right, so would anyone be interested in coming together to develop a consensus statement? There was a resounding yes to the question, so that was the next phase of the project.

Like my position statement, it was very easy to reach agreement as to what the statement needed to say, and after a few rounds of iterations we were nearly there. All apart from one group: the unions. The unions were reluctant to sign something that said that work was good for you. For the Faculty group leading the project, this was a blow. The strength and value of the statement lay in consensus—to have a position where government, employers, unions, and health professionals were all agreeing on something was pretty unique! To have the unions *not* involved somehow sent out a message that there was something missing, something wrong in what we were saying. It also meant that the most important group of all were not represented: the workers.

I met with Helen Kelly, the president of the New Zealand Council of Trades Unions (NZCTU, commonly known as the CTU). She told me that their concern was not the principle that work is good for health, but what about *bad* work? She said that they had union members who were injured or made ill by the work and then had to go back into the same work environment that made them unwell in the first instance.

As a doctor specializing in the health of workers, I had been in many, many different workplaces. I knew exactly what she was referring to—to be honest, you can spot a bad workplace a mile off, by the way they treat their workers. I agreed with her. I also agreed that things need to change. We agreed that working together was the best way to change things. Ultimately, we changed the title of the consensus statement to reflect this, to reflect the need for work to be *good work*. Helen Kelly went out on a limb to bring the unions along, and they became signatories. Helen herself became one of the greatest advocates for the health benefits of good work, and we presented together at several meetings.

It is important that I pause at this point, to acknowledge the late Helen Kelly, who was dearly loved in New Zealand. Helen was a passionate advocate for the health of workers. Sadly, although she was a non-smoker herself, she was diagnosed with lung cancer. She campaigned fiercely for improved safety in dangerous industries like forestry, and also for the right to die with dignity, right up to her death in October 2016.

Having completed the consensus statement, together with its list of signatories from government, employers, unions, and healthcare professionals (see Appendix 2), we set about organizing the launch. Some of the key concepts which underpinned the principles of the *Health Benefits of Good Work* came from the UK work of Professor Dame Carol Black. One of the working party pointed out that we needed someone like Dame Carol to launch the statement, as one of the world's foremost authorities on the relationship between health and work. I said, 'So why don't we ask Dame Carol?' When my colleagues stopped laughing, they suggested if I thought it was such a good idea, I should ask her. So I did.

Of course, she said yes. She would be happy to.

Dame Carol Black was the UK's first National Director of Health and Work. She was appointed by the government and asked to undertake a review of the health of the UK's working age population. This was subsequently published as the report *Working for a Healthier Tomorrow*, commonly (and eponymously) known as the 'Black Review'.[7] In it, she pointed out that the UK system for people going off sick was fundamentally flawed. People would go off work with an illness or injury (usually with an expectation that they would recover and go back to work) but many of them would simply remain on a long-term sickness benefit. After 23 months of absence from work, there was a 90 per cent chance that they would not return to work in the foreseeable future. She pointed out that the system failed people by not providing rehabilitation services and instead left them floundering at home, costing the country £100 billion per year.

One of the root causes of the failing of the system was the way that people were signed off work, with a medical certificate or 'sick note'. Even the title of this document was sending the wrong message. People were being labelled as sick, and were therefore assumed unable to work, and that was the way it remained. She recommended a change of mindset, from 'sick note' to 'fit note'. Instead of certifying that someone was fully unfit for work, the medical certificate should certify their capacity for work: what they were capable of doing at work, and therefore what restrictions would enable them to return to work. Along with this, she highlighted the need for training of GPs, as being central to the delivery of this new principle.

The concept was accepted by the government and brought into law in 2009. Sadly, the training for GPs was slow in coming and the uptake was initially low. The format of the form was such that it was possible for GPs to use it in the same way as the old sick note, and simply certify someone as being unfit for work. When Dame Carol reviewed the introduction of the fit note 2 years later, she found that many of the certificates were being used in this way, and that unfortunately the concept was not the initiator of positive change that it should have been.[8]

The launch of the consensus statement took place in Wellington in March 2011. The event was opened for the government, as a signatory, by the Minister Responsible for ACC, the Honourable Nick Smith. Helen Kelly spoke for the unions, Paul Mackay for Business New Zealand, and Dr Don Campbell for the Royal New Zealand College of General Practitioners.

At the launch, Dame Carol, who had been a rheumatologist and was also a past president of the Royal College of Physicians of London, said, 'If I have one regret from my years of practice as a rheumatologist, it is that I did not enquire about the patient's job. I didn't ask him or her what they did for a living, or even if they were still working.' She strongly emphasized the role of doctors in helping people to return to work—that returning to work is actually part of treatment and recovery of function for life. She said, 'Doctors have a clear duty and responsibility to make this happen and key roles to play. This begins with the necessary shifts in belief and understanding and reversing the belief that we have to be totally fit and well to return to work or that recovery from illness or injury must be total before return. Return to work must be considered a clinical goal.'

For most of us, work is a fundamental part of who we are. It's part of what defines us and gives meaning and connections in our lives. Yet, in many countries, we are now seeing generations for whom this is not true. They, like their parents, have never worked, and instead live lives of benefit dependency.

One of the factors that influences this situation positively or negatively is the doctors who provide medical certification. For some doctors, the connection between health and work is still not obvious. Certainly, that is the evidence from the UK. Unpublished work from New Zealand suggests that a higher proportion of GPs in New Zealand are aware of the health benefits of good work, and see encouraging and supporting people to return to work as part of their role.[9]

Why would this be? Doctors are very caring people who go into the profession to help people. For most it's a vocation. From my own experiences of thousands of cases where people haven't got back to work when we would have expected them to, and from looking back at my own training, I think the root causes lie both in the training of doctors and in the definition of health. I will explain this further in Chapter 3.

Why is this important for you to know? Because, to a significant extent, our health and wellbeing are influenced by the understanding of what we expect from our doctors and are told by them. At least, this used to be the case. Times are changing, and health and wellbeing is now an industry generating $4 trillion per year worldwide. It speaks of a very different model of health and functionality in life. It describes ways of improving health and getting the most out of lives, including our lives at work. It aspires to helping us 'be the best we can be'. Also, in this Information Age, the knowledge that used to provide the power differential between doctors and patients has been significantly eroded. The advent of 'Doctor Google', and an increasing desire for people to understand more about their own health and wellbeing, have changed that dramatically, even since I was a GP.

Does a doctor stating, about a 38-year-old with a partner and three children, that they are best remaining a long-term beneficiary, equate to empowering them to be 'the best they can be'? Not in my book.

Doctors are constrained by the system that they are working under. I understand that, in the UK, GP appointments are now on average nearly 10 minutes long (six per hour), rather than the 7½ (eight per hour) I worked to in the 1990s. How can a doctor be expected to manage disease and health and wellbeing and be concerned whether or not you are working and functioning fully in your life in 10 minutes? They can't.

Later in this book I will explain about calls for the average appointment length to increase to 15 minutes in the UK by 2030. How much difference is that likely to make?

The possibility is that doctors are more and more becoming experts in disease management at the same time that their patients are starting to focus on health and wellbeing. The opportunity is for the doctors who do want to work differently to take on the role of enablers of health and wellbeing, in partnership with their patients. We will always need doctors to be experts in disease management, but suddenly there is the opportunity for some doctors to work alongside patients to develop their health and wellbeing in a way which focuses on the prevention of ill health and disease. From what I'm hearing and reading, that is exactly what people are now looking for.

3

The Art of Medicine

From the age of 11, I knew I was going to be a doctor. It wasn't that I wanted to be a doctor, I just *knew*. I've heard a lot of people say that. That's why careers in the caring professions are sometimes referred to as a calling. They are certainly a vocation. Quite why, I couldn't have articulated, but I was fascinated by science and the human body, and I loved nature.

It was a huge advantage to me that my motivation to do well at school and be a straight-A student was very strong. I knew I had to work hard, because I knew the competition to get into medical school was intense.

On the first day of university, I walked up to the medical school building. Outside was a stone plaque. On it were engraved the words *Ars Longa Vita Brevis*.

I was puzzled; I didn't know what it meant. Oh, I knew how it translated, because I had done Latin at school. My mum told me I would need to do Latin to be a doctor. (I'm sure that was once true!) It translated as 'The art is long: life is short'.

That didn't compute with what I knew about medicine or with what I was going to learn. Medicine is a science, not an art. I was entering medicine in the heyday of medical science. There was a growing expectation that advances in medicine were going to cure modern diseases. If they hadn't already, it was just a matter of time.

Years later, I realized that the motto was an aphorism of Hippocrates, known as the 'Father of Western Medicine', even though he practised in Ancient Greece nearly 2500 years ago. Until Hippocrates, medicine had been very mystical. Hippocrates was the first known physician to consider the underlying cause of disease, the aetiology. He documented cases of illness to consider not only their possible underlying causes, but also their prognosis. What was the natural course of the condition?

Hippocrates decided that, in various illnesses, there were days of crisis, when either the patient would hit a turning point and start to recover, or deteriorate rapidly and perhaps die. His 'prescriptions' might have been medicines of the day, but often they weren't. He was a great proponent of rest, good

Positive Medicine. David Beaumont, Oxford University Press. © Oxford University Press 2021.
DOI: 10.1093/oso/9780192845184.003.0004

nutrition, and allowing the body to heal itself. He also introduced a code of ethics into medicine. His code covered the respect that doctors should show their teachers and their fellow doctors as well as the specifics of the rules by which they should engage with their patients. The Hippocratic oath, in evolved format, exists to this day and forms the basis for modern medical ethics.

If the basic tenet of the Hippocratic oath was 'First, do no harm', it can be said that the mantra of modern medicine is *First, do something.* The concept of 'watchful waiting' that I was taught at medical school, which came from Hippocrates, seems to have been replaced by an urgency to issue a perception or initiate investigations or interventions. This need to do something has been described as 'defensive medicine'. By doing something, the perception is that a doctor may avoid the accusation that they missed something or didn't treat something, but the reality is that it increases the chance they will make an error. The error rate in making a diagnosis is estimated to be between 10 and 20 per cent. *Doing something* greatly increases the chance of serious side effects from medication or intervention. It has been proposed that the third commonest cause of death in the US, after cardiovascular disease and cancer, is medical error.

The first 2 years of medicine for me were all about learning the science of medicine. Literally all. The three core subjects were anatomy, physiology, and biochemistry. On the very first day, I was introduced to my cadaver (a body that had been donated by a person, according to their wishes). One guy fainted. Nine out of the class of 150 students dropped out in that first week.

It's very different these days. My son, Matt, is a junior doctor. I recall with a smile on my face the call I received from him after his first day at medical school: 'Dad, you'll never believe it but we had a lecture from an orthopaedic surgeon and he brought in a real patient! I'm going to be an orthopaedic surgeon!' (He soon changed his mind about that.)

Today's medical training has patient contact threaded throughout the curriculum. Medical students are encouraged to consider what they are learning from the patient's perspective.

What does a doctor do?

My first clinical attachment, on a hospital ward, came in year 3. It was a general medicine ward. We had a teaching ward round with the consultant professor only a few weeks into my clinical training. He took us to see a man who had been admitted with a severe attack of asthma. He had been found to have abnormal blood and X-ray findings that wouldn't usually be found in asthma, including a very high result for a marker of inflammation, the erythrocyte sedimentation rate (ESR).

The consultant gathered us around the X-ray and asked me (I think I must have been the only student not looking at my shoes), 'What causes bronchospasm, fluffy opacities on chest X-ray, and an ESR greater than one hundred?'

I floundered to come up with a list of differential diagnoses that made any sense.

The consultant became exasperated with me, and said, in his lilting Welsh accent, 'Well it's polyarteritis nodosa, isn't it? You're a waste of space!'

As I reflect now, I realize that most doctors wouldn't have been able to come up with the diagnosis. There was no way I could have been expected to know such a rare condition, and asthma is an extremely rare manifestation of it. No, this was a great example of the ritual humiliation of medical students that has been portrayed so vividly in many films about the training of doctors. What purpose it serves I have no idea.

It was only in recent years that I watched the wonderful 1998 film *Patch Adams*, starring Robin Williams. Based on the life of Dr Hunter 'Patch' Adams, a maverick doctor who rebelled against the system, it tells the story of a young man who reached the lowest point in his life and stood on the brink of committing suicide. He realized the futility of suicide, and instead decided to go to medical school to make a difference in this world. His idealism is quickly shaken by what he experiences, and in rebelling against the system he puts on a red clown's nose and makes patients laugh.

At the end of the film, he makes his ultimate gesture of disrespect against the medical establishment, and establishes a place where patients can go for treatment with humanity and laughter, which he gives the pompous, medical-sounding name of The Gesundheit Institute. Gesundheit is merely the German word for health; it is also said when someone sneezes. That place of loving healing for patients still functions today, and Dr Adams remains a powerful advocate for compassion in medicine.

In the film, the students are welcomed to the medical school with a rousing opening address from the dean.

'Our job is to rigorously and ruthlessly train the humanity out of you and make you into something better. We're gonna make doctors out of you!'

Like me, early in his training, Patch goes on the consultant ward round with his fellow students. The consultant takes them to the bedside of a woman whose black toe is sticking out from under the sheets. He describes the presence of diabetes and advanced peripheral vascular disease leading to gangrene.

'It will have to come off. Any questions?'

The students all look at their shoes. Patch pushes his way to the front and says, quietly, 'Yes sir. What's her name?'

The consultant looks flustered. He clearly has no idea. (It is with shame I acknowledge that when I was a junior doctor we would refer to 'the cholecystitis in bed 3' and 'the pneumonia in bed 5', rather than referring to the patients by name.)

The underlying premise of the film is repeated several times:

We need to start treating the patient as well as the disease.

Our job is improving the quality of life, not just delaying death.

You treat a disease, you win, you lose. You treat a person; I'll guarantee you'll win.

Surely, *surely*, this is the vision of medicine (primary care specifically) in 2030 that is painted for doctors and patients by the RCGP in the UK in *Fit for the Future*, its 2019 vision statement.

The delivery of relationship-based, whole-person care will be at the heart of general practice. GPs will have more time to care for those patients with the most complex needs and will work with extended practice teams to provide enhanced continuity of care.

Patients will have more choice over the length, time and method of consultation. The standard face-to-face consultation length will be at least 15 minutes and more consultations will be delivered remotely through digital and video channels. GPs will have access to a wider range of data sources and diagnostic tools, and shared decision-making with patients will be the norm.[1]

Isn't it sad that the 'old way', as they describe it, is so entrenched in the system that they see it will take until 2030 to get to the 'new way'?

In the film, Patch says, 'I wanted to train to become a doctor so I could serve others'.

I did too. I believe that to be the case for most aspiring doctors who enter medical training. I believe that most doctors now would love to work to this aspiration: their purpose, their calling.

But the healthcare systems we work in don't allow it, or even, dare I say, even encourage it.

I have huge optimism for the future. When I talked to my son, Matt, about his medical training in New Zealand, he told me that the medical training curriculum changed a few years ago to become overtly patient centred. Medical students are taught the principles of compassion and empathy, and to consider the patient's perspective in everything they do. The New Zealand doctors of the future will start out with the same values and beliefs as Patch.

But what I didn't know when I was going through medical school was that doctors and their medical practice were already under attack. There was a growing discontent that the wonders of medical science were not all they were cracked up to be. That the amazing results that medical science was proclaiming were illusionary. Worse, that they were actually harming patients: not only by treatments, but also by the medicalization of society—a growing dependence on doctors to prescribe for conditions that are simply the experience of life and death. A better way was being proposed.

In his 1974 book, *Medical Nemesis*, Ivan Illich described the increasing realization and evidence that modern medicine, and doctors specifically, were harming people, and that doctors' effectiveness was 'an illusion'.[2] He called this effect 'iatrogenesis', which he defines as 'doctor made'. The term has now come into common usage in the healthcare literature to mean 'inadvertent harm caused by doctors'.

Illich used the phrase 'medical nemesis' in his title. A nemesis is the 'inescapable cause of one's own downfall'. His opening sentence sets out his thesis:

The medical establishment has become a major threat to health.[3]

Illich argued that the medical system, and the medical model that doctors practise to, was flawed—so flawed, that it would itself become the inescapable cause of the downfall of modern medicine. So inevitable was the downfall, in his opinion, that he predicted that 'The health professions are on the brink of an unprecedented housecleaning campaign'.[4]

It's been a long time coming, but from what the RCGP in the UK is saying, that time may be now.

Illich described three levels of harm. The first is what he termed 'clinical iatrogenesis', the harms arising from medical error, over-prescribing, and drug side effects causing serious complications and death. The second level he calls 'social iatrogenesis'—the social role played by doctors to label people as sick, including certification of absence from work, and thereby creating a 'sick' society and a dependency on doctors that is legitimized by doctors. This is also reflected in the work of Dame Carol Black and the 'sick note'. The third level he calls 'cultural iatrogenesis'; perhaps the most insidious and subtle of all.

He accuses doctors of medicalizing normal life experiences such as birth and death, and thereby robbing people of the ability to cope with life. He persuasively describes iatrogenesis as medical intervention that cripples 'personal responses to pain, disability, impairment, anguish, and death'.[5]

In the film *Patch Adams*, Patch has something to say in agreement with this last point: 'What's wrong with death, sir? What are we so mortally afraid of? Why can't we treat death with a certain amount of humility and dignity, and decency, and God forbid, even humour. Death is not the enemy, gentlemen. If you're going to fight a disease, let's fight one of the most terrible diseases of all: indifference.'

Perhaps the indifference that Patch is referring to is indifference to the challenges that Ivan Illich raised so persuasively. What if the medical establishment in the 1970s got it horribly wrong and did more harm than good. Isn't it indifference to turn our backs to that possibility?

In New Zealand and Australia, the RACP, the professional body of all 25,000 specialist doctors and specialists in training, is not turning its back. Its EVOLVE initiative is systematically researching the many different treatments and interventions that are commonly used and prescribed in every medical speciality and for which there is no evidence of efficacy, or only scanty evidence, or for which the risk of side effects exceeds the benefits.

Perhaps one of the most scandalous examples of harm caused by doctors is the opioid epidemic (also called the opioid crisis) that is sweeping the Western world. Escalating numbers of people dying from opioid overdoses, mostly unintended, with significant numbers associated with opioids prescribed by doctors for chronic pain. In 2018, there were nearly 70,000 deaths in the US alone.[6]

In May 2019, in a session of the annual congress of the RACP, the former President of the Chapter of Addiction Medicine, Dr Adrian Reynolds (a specialist doctor in the management of addiction), spoke about the problem in a session entitled 'The opioid epidemic—iatrogenesis on a global scale'. He explained that the evidence for the prescribing of opioids in non-cancer pain is weak, but the evidence that the risks outweigh the benefits is very strong. The position of the RACP is therefore that opioids should not be prescribed for non-cancer chronic pain.

The contribution of doctors to the opioid epidemic is completely unnecessary and avoidable.

In the same session, a colleague of mine, Dr Chris Rumball, an occupational physician and pain specialist, explained the principles of modern pain management. Both he and I spend clinical time with patients helping them withdraw from inappropriately prescribed opioids. He explained that not only is there only weak evidence for their efficacy, but there is good evidence that opioids can actually aggravate the body's response to pain.

Modern pain management is based on a multidisciplinary team approach to help people understand their pain and learn to self-manage and get on with their lives despite pain.

Illich's solution? A society in which input from doctors is kept to the minimum necessary to sustain the health of that society, a society in which the focus is on health, but health defined in a very different way to that defined by doctors. (I will address this more fully in Chapter 4.) The shift of focus is from illness management to improving health and preventing ill health.

In doing so, the responsibility for health moves to the individual and the society that they live in:

> That society which can reduce professional intervention to the minimum will provide the best conditions for health. The greater the potential for autonomous adaptation to self, to others, and to the environment, the less management of adaptation will be needed or tolerated.[7]

In other words, the more control that people have over their own lives and can adapt to the changing circumstances that their life journey brings, the healthier they will be. Return to life, return to health!

Illich reached the conclusion that the key to health is in supporting people to address a concept that I will address shortly, the social determinants of health:

> Healthy people are those who live in healthy homes on a healthy diet in an environment equally fit for birth, growth, work, healing, and dying; they are sustained by a culture that enhances the conscious acceptance of limits to population, of aging, of incomplete recovery and ever-imminent death. Healthy people need minimal bureaucratic interference to mate, give birth, share the human condition, and die.[8]

Over 40 years ago, Illich succinctly predicted the crisis in primary care that has now hit the UK. The RCGP's vision for general practice in the UK by 2030, in all honesty, barely touches the sides of the solution proffered by Illich. The problem has been created by a system that generates people's dependence on doctors. The solution does not lie in making those doctors more accessible. Instead, it lies in demedicalization of the events and consequences of normal life and empowering and educating people to take control over their own life and health.

A new model of medical practice

There were other visionaries in the 1970s who reached the same conclusions as Illich—that medicine as practised by doctors was far from the solution, indeed it was a significant part of the problem.

Dr John Powles, in a paper written in 1973 entitled 'On the limitations of modern medicine',[9] presented similar problems to Illich, and similar solutions. He pointed out that there had developed an accepted dogma that the solutions to society's ills lay in modern medicine and doctors. But he pointed out that the direction that medicine went from that point on was a matter of choice for society. He identified two possibilities: '[T]here have always been two conflicting approaches within medicine—one emphasising the potency of clinical intervention (the "engineering approach"), the other emphasising the importance of way of life factors (the "ecological approach")'.[10]

Powles felt the arguments for change were so strong that this must inevitably be accepted as necessary (a far more optimistic belief in the insight of mankind than the nemesis seen by Illich): 'With a rising proportion of illness evidently man-made, and increasing restrictions on the further increase of resource consumption for medical care, medicine does seem bound to move in an "ecological" direction'. The 'ecological' direction he saw was prevention. It was health and wellbeing. It was empowerment and self-responsibility.

It hasn't happened.

Another person who saw that things must change, and how they should change, was Dr George Engel. His seminal 1977 *Science* paper, 'The need for a new medical model: a challenge for biomedicine', has had far more impact than the others mentioned.[11] His 'biopsychosocial model', over 40 years later, forms the basis for the understanding of work disability and underpins most of modern rehabilitation practice. It's the model that occupational physicians like myself are taught as part of our training, and also the many allied health professionals who work in rehabilitation: nurses, physiotherapists, occupational therapists, and psychologists. It's a multidisciplinary model.

But the majority of doctors don't work to it, and at the presentations I give to groups of doctors, often half of the attendees haven't heard of it.

All medical students in New Zealand are taught it, and therefore all qualified younger doctors. However, a senior medical registrar recently explained to me, 'The biopsychosocial model is taught to us throughout our training. But when we get to the wards the senior doctors haven't even heard of it, so the theory goes out of the window and never becomes practice.'

I'm honestly not surprised. Although the paper was written, and the model described, before my training, I was not taught it at medical school. Nor were other doctors of my generation, I suspect, or for many years following.

The rationale for a new model of practice to be proposed came from Dr Engel's own experience as a clinician. He was a very interesting doctor in that he was dual qualified as both a psychiatrist and physician. In the latter role, he worked in the fields of gastroenterology and neurology. He found that in both clinics there were many patients with significant symptoms and disability for which no underlying cause could be found. All tests were negative. This completely went against the principles of the medical model, which presupposes that if there are symptoms, then it is only a matter of identifying the underlying pathology and you can treat the conditions. But there were many patients presenting to his clinics with medically unexplained symptoms.

As he went around medical conferences and listened to discussions about this conundrum, he realized that what he was hearing was wrong. It dismissed these patients and left them with no medical care. He realized that the problem was the very model by which the doctors are trained, the medical model. He saw the underlying premise on which doctors work had created a crisis of care:

> Medicine's crisis stems from the logical inference that since 'disease' is defined in terms of somatic [physical] parameters, physicians need not be concerned with psychosocial issues which lie outside medicine's responsibility and authority.[12]

This was exactly my experience when I encountered a doctor who felt that helping someone back to work was not their responsibility. It has been confirmed in the research of Professor Debbie Cohen and Sir Mansel Aylward, which found that 'General Practitioners felt their role was to provide support and management of health-related issues only and the management of long-term worklessness lay outside of their role.'[13]

Worse still were the attitudes towards this 'problem' from some of the colleagues whom Engel quoted:

> One authority urged that medicine 'concentrate on the "real" diseases and not get lost in the psychosocial underbrush ...'. ... Another participant called for 'a disentanglement of the organic elements of disease from the psychosocial elements of human malfunction', arguing that medicine should deal with the former only.[14]

This incredibly pompous and judgemental position relegated patients with medically unexplained symptoms to being nothing to do with the doctor or modern medicine, and left them labelled as problem or 'heartsink' patients.

The biopsychosocial model works on an understanding that only a small percentage of our health is related to purely physical (bio-) factors (perhaps 20–30 per cent). The remainder are due to due to the influence of life, lifestyle, and environmental factors (psychosocial). Therefore, these are the factors that explain illness and disease. These are the influences of the social determinants of health.

The medical model, by deciding to ignore psychosocial factors, takes doctors out of the equation for influencing the social determinants of health and the associated illness. Only if someone develops a disease with clear underlying pathology does the medical model doctor need to be involved—as an expert in disease management. No wonder patients with so-called medically unexplained symptoms are so unhappy about how they are perceived and treated by some doctors. Medically unexplained symptoms are unexplained by the medical model, but they're not unable to be explained.

Here's a parody of my 6 years of training to be a doctor: the medical model in one paragraph. Patient comes to doctor and describes symptoms; doctor takes a 'history', examines, requests investigations, reaches a diagnosis, and prescribes treatment. If that works, then the patient is satisfied, and the doctor feels s/he has done a good job. If it doesn't, the patient comes back, the doctor enquires further about the symptoms, examines, investigates, and revises diagnosis and treatment. If that works, that's great; both are still satisfied. If it doesn't, the patient returns, dissatisfied. The doctor then has three choices. She or he can go around the loop again, refer to specialist hospital outpatients, or 'monitor'. 'Come back in 3 months and we'll see if it is improved.' Both are left dissatisfied.

A parody, maybe, but one which I'm sure has been experienced by every doctor and every patient. I'm sure you can identify with it, whichever side of that (artificial) divide you're on, doctor or patient.

Society expects doctors to make a diagnosis and prescribe treatment. It's very hard for doctors not to live up to that expectation. Sometimes it feels as though patients believe we have omnipotence in finding solutions to life problems that have been medicalized, or even medical problems that patients expect to be prescribed for yet doctors don't feel are appropriate.

The simplest example from my general practice was antibiotic prescribing for viral upper respiratory tract illness (coughs and colds). It had been drummed into me during training that you only prescribe antibiotics where there is good evidence of a bacterial infection which is likely to respond to the relevant antibiotic. There are very good reasons for this: avoiding side effects of medication and development of antibiotic allergy and resistance in the individual, and development of widespread antibiotic resistance in the community, which is now happening worldwide. Yet, because as a young doctor I often did not prescribe when the patient expected me to (sometimes demanded!), I had many patients express their dissatisfaction, often vehemently.

Criticisms of the medical model have focused on its being a reductionist model: that it has been simplified so far that it has lost its utility. The underlying premise inherent in the loop of the medical model (that symptoms = pathology = diagnosis) creates four problems:

1. The concept that there must be a diagnosis to explain symptoms creates the dichotomy that therefore there either is a treatment or there isn't. If there is no 'treatment' once a diagnosis is reached, the doctor can say, 'Sorry, there's nothing more I can do for you. There's no treatment.'

2. The patient is taken out of the context of their life. They are reduced to a diagnosis (the psychosocial factors are automatically discounted as not being the responsibility of the doctor).

3. What about medically unexplained symptoms? Since no pathology has been identified and yet there is pressure to reach a diagnosis, the symptoms are collected together and a descriptive diagnosis given, but one that sounds justifiably 'medical'. Thus, if a patient presents with widespread pain, tenderness in the muscles over a wide area of the body, together with other symptoms associated with disability, they may be given a diagnosis of fibromyalgia. Fibromyalgia is word coined by doctors from a Greek root. It is a symptom description for 'pain in the muscles and fibrous tissue'. It comes from an era when doctors commonly used Greek- or Latin-derived words to name symptoms, such as low back pain being given the pseudo-diagnostic label of 'lumbago'. The cynic would say it was to perpetuate the power imbalance between doctor and patient.

4. Further, if no pathology has been identified and the patient is referred for specialist opinion, then it is very likely that no pathology will be identified by that specialist either. This perpetuates patient dissatisfaction, and increases the likelihood that further, more invasive investigations will be initiated—yet still no diagnosis is reached. In busy specialist clinics, this often leads to very brief and unsatisfactory consultations, ending either with the advice that no cause can be found, or referral on to another

specialist: 'All your gastrointestinal investigations are negative. Let's rule out a gynaecological cause.'

The doctor and psychoanalyst Michael Balint called this fourth circumstance 'the collusion of anonymity'. It is ultimate doctor buck-passing. We don't know what it is or what to do, so let's give the problem to someone else. Balint set up support groups for doctors to bring such challenging cases to. He helped GPs explore what underlying events in a person's life may be contributing to or causing the illness. These 'Balint groups' continue to the present in some places. It was Balint also who proposed that the commonest drug prescribed in general practice 'was the doctor himself' (the male pronoun was always used in the 1950s and 1960s, when Balint wrote).[15]

This concept of 'the drug doctor' is important. The care of doctors is a highly effective treatment, but like all drugs, it too can have side effects. Predictions made by doctors can be seen as gospel, and a statement such as 'You'll never work again' becomes a self-fulfilling prophesy.

It may be that the inability of the medical model to explain 'medically un-explained symptoms' is the biggest flaw of all. I will explore it further in a later chapter. In human cost, and cost to the healthcare system, the implications of this problem are enormous. It is estimated that around 30 per cent, and possibly as high as 50 per cent, of consultations with GPs are for medically unexplained symptoms.[16] Because many of them are referred for specialist assessment, the same percentage is found in secondary care, specialist clinics.[17] The degree of human suffering and impact on healthcare delivery cannot be overstated.

Like Dr George Engel, Dr Mark Lane (a former president of the RACP) is a gastroenterologist. Of the many different medically unexplained symptoms (affecting every part and system of the body), irritable bowel syndrome is one of the better understood in terms of the underlying mechanisms and linkage with life events. Mark Lane told me that often half his time in outpatient clinics is spent explaining to patients that they *don't* need an endoscopy (a fibreoptic scope inserted either into the oesophagus or rectum), because he is confident that the test will be normal and therefore unnecessary risk would be involved in performing it. Instead, he spends time with them exploring what has been going on in their lives.

Dr Jonathan Christiansen, another former New Zealand president of the RACP, is a cardiologist. He told me that half of the patients he sees for investi-gation of possible heart problems have normal results and are diagnosed with 'non-cardiac chest pain', a medically unexplained symptom. He recounted a story of a man he had seen in clinic and had just informed he had negative test results. The man said, 'You know, they've made me redundant. After all these years. Without a thank you or an acknowledgement of what I've done for that company.' Jonathan could see his pain. His chest pain was a manifestation of the distress and loss of meaning he felt at a major transition in his life.

I believe that the art of medicine is applying the science in the context of a person's whole life. I believe there are many doctors who feel the same as I do, and practise with that intent to the extent that the system allows (which gives little room for them to do so), just as Mark Lane and Jonathan Christiansen do.

As I talk to people about their health and wellbeing and the role of doctors, I have many people say to me, 'I've got the best doctor in the world'. I'm sure they do.

4

What Are 'Health and Wellbeing'?

I was running a workshop on health and wellbeing for the senior management team of a power distribution company. They had asked me to undertake a review of the health and wellbeing of their staff: office workers and the power-line workers in the field. I started with the basics. I asked them, 'What is the definition of health?'

Within a few seconds, the IT manager said, 'Everything working correctly'. What a succinct description!

I said, 'That's a great summary of what I was taught about the definition at medical school.'

I showed them the definition of health that I had retrieved from an online dictionary: 'Health is the condition of being well or free from disease.'

This is the definition of health that is the underlying principle of the medical model: that once a doctor has identified a disease process and treated it, then she has helped the patient achieve health. As patients, it is also what we have come to expect from our interactions with doctors, and is therefore our default definition of health.

The human resources manager said, 'I think health is bigger than that. For me, health is about being able to enjoy special time with my husband and have the energy to play with my kids.'

I agreed with her. That had been exactly my realization after my heart attack. I had made a complete recovery physically, but I didn't feel I had 'health'. How can we capture that to define what health truly is?

I ran a series of workshops with the field workers, at their bases in rural New Zealand. I asked them what they thought about their health.

One of them said, 'Do we look healthy?'

They all laughed. They were all men, mostly 50-plus, and, to be honest, were obviously overweight and didn't look very fit. One of them made a more serious comment that I found very insightful. He said:

> You know, when you're in your 20s, you've come from that time in your life when you've done some sport, and maybe carried on with it, and you're pretty

Positive Medicine. David Beaumont, Oxford University Press. © Oxford University Press 2021.
DOI: 10.1093/oso/9780192845184.003.0005

fit and healthy. In your 30s you get all wrapped up with life, but it's OK, your body seems to cope with it and look ok. In your 40s it all starts to catch up with you. We let ourselves go; and by the time we get into our 50s it's too late to do anything about it.

I asked them about seeing their doctors. They confirmed what we know about middle-aged men. 'We only go to a doctor if there's something wrong.' This demographic is at once the most at risk and the worst for health-seeking behaviour. They don't see their doctor until a disease event has taken place. Often it's too late.

The company has invested a lot in the health and wellbeing of their workers, including a holistic health app. I asked them what they thought of it. Much laughter ensued. 'It started out with a hiss and a roar at the launch meeting 2 years ago. It's really airy-fairy. We get a weekly email telling us what stuff we should be doing. I think most of us just delete it without reading it. I know I do.'

That was really interesting, because the national health and safety manager for one of the major banks had called me only a few weeks earlier to say that that they had introduced a health and wellbeing app for their staff 2 years ago, but only 20 per cent of them were using it, and it seemed to be the 20 per cent who were already looking after their health. He sent me an article he had just read in the national press, which said that a big research study in the US, undertaken by the University of Illinois, had concluded that health and wellbeing programmes in the workplace don't work.

This flew in the face of conventional wisdom and what I knew of other research, so it was worth looking into.

I read the study report from the research team at the University of Illinois. It was a very big study, which appeared sound. They had introduced programmes for the employees of the university, at significant cost, and undertaken the research to try to demonstrate an improvement in the health and wellbeing of the staff and financial savings in healthcare costs. The interventions achieved neither.

Economic evaluations of this nature are relatively easy to perform in the US compared to other countries, because employers are responsible for the healthcare costs of their workers. The programmes to improve health and wellbeing were not found to change healthy behaviours in their workers, and therefore made no difference to the university's healthcare costs. This was confusing to me, because I knew of research, including in Australia, that found that investing in the health and wellbeing of employees had improved engagement, reduced staff turnover, and increased productivity. Research showed that every $1 spent on workers' health resulted in a $3 increase in profit from increased productivity.

To investigate this apparently contradictory finding, I asked a senior American occupational physician, Dr Ray Fabius. Ray has researched extensively on the business case for investing in the health of workers. He explained that, in order for health and wellbeing programmes to be effective, there is one essential prerequisite: they only work in the presence of a 'culture of health'. As I understand the principle, a culture of health exists in an organization where the health of its workforce is an *overt* priority of the organization. I'm sure that's often the intent, but it's not obvious to the workers. A culture of health needs to be led from the top of the organization, with values and policies set (and modelled) by the board and senior management, with the health and wellbeing of workers an explicitly stated priority. Workers are clear that they are seen and respected as individuals with value to the organization, and it is also acknowledged that they have families for whom they play important roles.

Dr Ray Fabius is an influential thought-leader who provides advice to many of America's top companies. He provides a persuasive argument that the workplace is a key setting to influence the health of the population. And the way to do it is by impacting lifestyle and life choices and addressing the social determinants of health. We're not going to achieve that merely by checking blood pressure and measuring cholesterol in people's lunch hour at work. To achieve this, a bigger definition of health is needed.

What is health?

In 1946, the World Health Organization (WHO) defined health in its founding constitution. This august body had already identified that the medical view of health was deficient. The WHO defined health as:

> A state of complete physical, mental and social well-being and not merely the absence of disease or infirmity.[1]

I was taught this definition at medical school, but it meant nothing to me then. It was impossible for me to conceptualize what this meant against what I was being taught about the role of doctors. In recent years, the WHO definition has been criticized on a number of levels. Key to the criticism is, first, that while it is clearly appropriate to develop a broader definition of what health is, the broader the definition, the more it changes with time. Health is not a 'state': it is a dynamic, changing process. If we look at our psychological health, then our state of mind changes every day. In fact, even from a physical perspective, although there is a definition of the difference between a normal blood pressure and an abnormal one, the fact is that our blood pressure fluctuates greatly through the course of a day. From a social perspective, our social circumstances change through life, and even the journey of life includes the passage of time and the fact that we age, and our health changes with time. So, the definition needs to include the concept that health is a dynamic process. Second, what is 'a state of complete physical, mental and social wellbeing'? Am I in that state now? No. Are you in that state now? Probably not. By definition, a person with a disability can never be in that state. Therefore, as a tool for understanding our own health, and for developing models of medical practice, it is unworkable.

In March 2003, *The Lancet*, one of the most respected medical journals in the world, published an editorial proposing a new definition of health as 'the ability to adapt'. It saw this definition moving beyond the perfection required by the WHO definition, and beyond the concept that science was going to eradicate human suffering (as it clearly hasn't). By defining health for an individual as being the ability to adapt, it took into account the need to adapt to illness, to pain, to suffering, to ageing, and to changes in life circumstances; in other words, the life events that happen inevitably to us all. *The Lancet* proposed that this new definition would allow doctors to transcend the complexities of disease to see the patient in the context of what was happening in their lives 'and offer a very practical mission for modern medicine'. In this paradigm, 'health is defined not by the doctor, but by the person, according to his or her functional needs. The role of the doctor is to help the individual adapt to their unique prevailing condition. This should be the meaning of "personalised medicine" ... It puts the individual patient, not the doctor, in a position of self-determining authority to define his or her health needs. The doctor becomes a partner in delivering those needs.'

Later that year, in response to the editorial in *The Lancet*, a conference of 40 invited international experts considered the definition of health from a healthcare, social, and patient perspective. They concluded that it was indeed time to move beyond the WHO definition, for health to be viewed as a dynamic process, and the definition to include the ability to adapt. It was also agreed that a key concept was the patient's own ability to self-manage, and that the social determinants of health were important factors that must be included. They did not reach a definite consensus on the definition.

In 2011, one of the conference participants, Dr Machteld Huber, published in *The BMJ* the proposal that the new unified definition should be that 'health is the ability to adapt and self-manage in the face of social, physical, and emotional challenges'.[2] I would like to propose that we shorten that definition:

Health is the ability to adapt and self-manage in the face of life's challenges.

Dr Huber went on to research the acceptability of the definition with various stakeholders in the Netherlands: patients and citizens, healthcare providers, policymakers, researchers, and insurers. The resulting outcomes were broad agreement as to the acceptability and utility of the definition, although with different emphases as to the components that would make up the domains of this more inclusive and patient-centred definition of health. Some 32 different aspects of a person's life were brought together into six different categories:

Bodily functions
Mental functions and perception
Spiritual/existential dimension
Quality of life
Social and societal participation
Daily functioning.[3]

For patients, the importance of each of these six domains was relatively equal—in other words, patients thought that 'health' should encompass all of these areas to address their needs. Policymakers had the greatest variation from the other stakeholders, and gave the greatest range of scores across the different domains. Basically, they scored bodily functions and the physical domain as the highest, and the other five domains significantly lower—very significantly lower than any other group. Since policymakers are the people who define healthcare systems and the priorities which drive them, there may be a clue here as to why our healthcare systems are so physically focused and why the medical model predominates.

Dr Huber's intention was to do the preliminary groundwork towards the operationalization of the definition, turning it from theory to practice, to a model of practice that doctors could work to in the new, 'patient-centred' approach. Since she noted that patients ranked all six domains as being of similar importance, the next part of the research was to look at how these domains were prioritized by healthcare professionals: doctors, nurses, and physiotherapists. Interestingly, the relative importance given to each domain by nurses was almost identical to that of the patients. Doctors rated the importance of the spiritual and social participation domains lower than patients, with physiotherapists falling between the two. When I talked to nurse colleagues, they were not surprised, since all these domains form an integral part of their training.

This means that all six domains will need to form part of the model of medical practice that operationalizes the new definition of health, if it is to truly address the needs of patients and place them at the centre of the process (to be 'patient centred').

One thing I need to make clear at this point: 'spiritual' in this context does not equate to religion. The constituent components making up the spiritual or existential domain included meaning in life, striving for aims or ideals, consideration of future prospects, and acceptance of what is. 'Spiritual' in this sense is about finding meaning in life—past, present, and future—and therefore is something we all have in common. I will explore this further in a later chapter.

Positive health

There was one further concept that Dr Huber concluded from this work: that operationalizing the new definition of health led to a view of health that is different to the old model. It can no longer be that to find 'health' means having the absence of disease. Finding health must be a bigger goal than this. Having health is a positive state, not the absence of a negative one. To distinguish the new way from the old way, she proposed the term 'positive health' to capture this concept.[4]

This is not the first time that the absence of disease, or illness, has been realized to be incomplete as a concept to deliver the full prospects for human potential. In the field of psychology, two visionaries reached the same conclusion: if we study the presence of disease or illness in people in order to identify treatments or management strategies to make them better, the end point can only go as far as the absence of disease. It settles for 'good enough'.

What if we were to start at the opposite end of the spectrum, not with people struggling with illness, but people who are seemingly thriving and living life to the fullest extent? The first visionary is Abraham Maslow, well known for the theory named after him, Maslow's hierarchy of needs, described in his paper 'A theory of human motivation', published in 1943.[5] The other is Professor Martin Seligman.

I recommend that you look up the TED talk by Professor Seligman, entitled 'The new era of positive psychology'.[6] In it he describes his realization that, for many years as a psychologist, he had spent many hours with clients with mental health conditions, trying, as he put it, 'to make miserable people less miserable'. Not only was psychology not particularly good at achieving this goal, but on the occasions he did successfully achieve relief of symptoms for clients, he did not find that they were actually happy at the end of the process. Basically, they were coping with life and no more.

In 1998, Seligman became president of the American Psychological Association. This was the platform he needed to shake the establishment with the proposal that psychology explore a new direction, a new science, that of positive psychology. This proposed that, rather than seeing the purpose of psychology as taking people who were suffering and getting them to the point of coping, that people who are coping can be helped to the point that they are flourishing in their lives.

Seligman immediately saw the connection between the concept of improving life satisfaction in this way and the idea that this resulted in happiness. He captured the concept in his 2002 book *Authentic Happiness.*[7] By 2011, he had realized that this was not sufficient, that his model had missed key pieces of the jigsaw. He corrected this in his book *Flourish: A Visionary New Understanding of Happiness and Wellbeing.*[8] Instead of wellbeing leading to happiness and life satisfaction, he realized that these are parts of the whole.

Attempts to define wellbeing have been limited by the realization that it cannot be captured by a string of words, since it has several different components to it. I recommend Professor Seligman's book *Flourish* not only as the best description of wellbeing I have found, but also for providing a review of the scientific evidence for the validity of developing the skills needed to flourish in our lives—and the associated benefits to our health.

Seligman defines wellbeing as having five components, which he captures under the acronym PERMA:

Positive emotion
Engagement
Relationships
Meaning
Achievement

Positive emotion includes the feelings that go with happiness, joy, contentment; the features that we easily think of when we consider our wellbeing. How happy are you? You can rate yourself against the hundreds of thousands of other people who have used the questionnaire on Professor Seligman's website (https://www.authentichappiness.sas.upenn.edu/).

Engagement is the process by which we become fully engrossed in something we enjoy doing or are particularly good at. It's those times when you're doing something so intently that time seems to stand still. It's been described as being in a state of 'flow'. Seligman points out that this is most likely to occur when we are doing the things that we are best at, most skilled at, and that align most closely with our signature strengths. Again, it's well worthwhile using the signature strengths questionnaire on his website to get a feel for what yours are.

Relationships in our lives are increasingly becoming an area of research. Positive relationships with our family and loved ones, our friends, and within our communities have all been clearly demonstrated to improve our lives and our health.

Meaning is about seeing ourselves as being part of, and contributing to, something bigger than ourselves. Leading lives with meaning and purpose has been found to be one of the greatest drivers for our lives. It's the beneficial effect that we have on other people through our thoughts and actions. In existential terms, that our life is worthwhile simply because we exist and impact other people's lives and make a positive difference (to many or even a few).

Achievement is a major human driver. Sometimes, it's good enough to achieve something for its own sake and not because it leads to anything else. But as humans, we enjoy creating, we enjoy the pleasure and self-satisfaction of a job well done. Seligman saw this as the fifth and integral component of wellbeing.

There is one further point I would draw your attention to here. As an occupational physician, my particular interest is the role of work in people's lives and health. Just look back at the list of those five components of our wellbeing. It is easy to see how all five can be found in a job which is fulfilling: a job which brings meaning to our life because of the contribution that we are making; that gives us a sense of accomplishment for a job well done; that gets us engrossed in tasks that we know we're good at (we might even think we are 'the best' at!); and that gives us social contact and relationships with our co-workers. In surveys of job satisfaction, I often find that the one thing that people highlight about their job is the people they work with, along with happiness and positive emotions. That may sound like an idealistic description to you, but it *does* happen, even if not all the time. It also forms a yardstick by which to check if your job measures up and what you might consider doing about it.

In *Flourish*, Professor Seligman examined the research into the effect of wellbeing on health. He found there is a clear relationship between wellbeing and improved health; specifically, a relationship between wellbeing and lower mortality from cardiovascular disease, cancer, and even all-cause mortality. He therefore proposes that future models of healthcare must include both health and wellbeing. He reached exactly the same conclusion as Dr Huber; namely, that this new understanding of health and wellbeing needs to be differentiated from the old model. He also proposed the term 'positive health' to distinguish this from the old way.

What's your 'why'?

As I've described, I've practised to the old way. As a GP, I tried to influence health by giving health promotion advice: 'Lose weight, stop smoking, cut down your alcohol.' My overwhelming feeling is that such advice has made little difference to people's healthy behaviours. If anything, it may have added to the sense of guilt that people feel because they intuitively know that they've overweight or unhealthy. Guilt is a very poor motivator; in fact, it demoralizes.

My thinking about how doctors can influence people to change behaviour changed dramatically a few years ago, when I watched a TED talk by the business guru Simon Sinek. In a video presentation which has been watched by millions of people, Simon Sinek tells us to 'Start with Why' (also the title of his book). He tells us that great leaders, and great companies, don't do what comes naturally to most people, which is to describe *what* needs to happen, *how* it can be done, and then, often as an afterthought, *why*. Instead, what they do first is to define the why. What is the purpose of this? Why will it make a difference? By defining the *why*, starting with *why*, to do it (whatever it may be) becomes an imperative. It has to happen. That leads on to *how* it can be achieved, and finally the specifics, the *what* details.

As I look at health promotion and prevention of disease, I realize that most of what doctors and the healthcare system do is tell people *what* to do (and only a tiny proportion of time and resource is spent even on doing that). Very rarely is information given as to *how* a patient could achieve the advice being given, and this (almost) never articulates the *why*. To say 'If you lose 15 kg, your blood pressure and cholesterol will come down, and we'll be able to reduce your diabetes drugs' is not a meaningful *why* in the context of the circumstances of a person's life. In fact, it's so generic that it is almost meaningless as a motivator.

So here is where health and wellbeing come together. If health is 'the ability to adapt and self-manage in the face of life's challenges', and wellbeing leads to the ability to flourish in life (an amazing and desirable aspiration), then surely, to achieve flourishing in our lives becomes our *why*. It becomes the goal, the motivator.

And there's evidence.

Maslow's hierarchy of needs, which I referred to earlier in this chapter, is a model for understanding human behaviour and motivation. Many people have heard of it. It's been used successfully by organizations and companies to understand the motivation of their workers and do their best to support and develop them. It is also widely referred to in the area of personal development.

The hierarchy of needs is usually displayed as a triangle with five tiers of needs, with the top tier, the pinnacle, being self-actualization (Fig. 4.1).[9] The underlying premise of the whole construct is that as human beings we share a desire, a drive, to become the best we can be. Self-actualization means to grow to become the person we were actually meant to be, the best version of ourselves. 'What a man can be, he must be', as Maslow put it. However, in order to achieve this pinnacle of self-fulfilment we have certain needs we must fulfil, at least to some degree.

The baseline tier, the basic need, Maslow describes as physiological. He explains that the body has an amazing ability to self-regulate, to keep parameters such as temperature, blood pressure, hydration, and blood chemistry (e.g. blood sugar) within a range of normality. This ability is known as *homeostasis*, literally, keeping within the same state. However, to do that the body has to have water, food, and sleep, and also be able to fulfil basic functions, such as sex for procreation. So thirst, hunger, sleepiness, and desire for sex are basic fundamental drives. Without fulfilling these, the person is not likely to be able to focus on anything else, and, at worst, does not survive.

Above this are the safety needs. In order to function properly, to focus on getting on with our lives, we need to feel safe in the environment we're in.

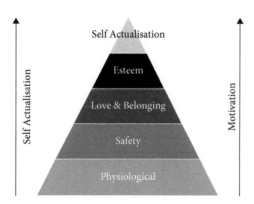

Fig. 4.1 Maslow's hierarchy of needs.

We need to have a roof over our heads, a place we call home in which we feel safe and protected. Our physiological needs are still important here, too—we need to know where our next meal is coming from. For this reason, poverty and work also come into play here—the safety of knowing we can pay our bills.

Maslow points out that nowhere in human existence is safety more important than childhood. Children, from babies and infants up, have a dominant need for safety. Much of that feeling of safety is provided by their environment and their parents. This need is so easily disturbed for children, and a lack of safety creates fear. In a state of fear, it is hard for children to develop and grow. Progression up the hierarchy of needs is limited, and things like learning and socialization suffer.

It is in this basic human need for safety that we find the social determinants of health: 'The conditions in which people are born, grow, live, work, and age.' Here also is the explanation for why childhood, and the first thousand days of life in particular, are fundamental in defining the shape of our lives and health, and the starting point for adult disease.

Above this, we have the need for love. Once our physiological and safety needs are met, we need to feel love—to love and be loved; and also to feel a sense of belonging—to the person we love, to the family, to our friends, and to the community we live in. Sex comes into this category too; not as a basic drive for procreation and satisfaction of a need, but as a reflection of our love.

If we have love and affection in our lives, then we are in a position where we can develop self-esteem and self-respect, and therefore esteem and respect for other people. So many people who have been through dysfunctional relationships where they have not felt loved, or have not been able to truly give love, whether within a family or in a love relationship, lack self-esteem and lose their self-respect. This need is about being able to love ourselves. Many people find it challenging.

Maslow points out that this pattern is not fixed, and will vary from person to person. But assuming some combination of having all these needs met, then the ultimate goal, and it is a shared goal, is to become self-actualized. Like Martin Seligman (over 50 years later), Maslow pointed out that to define what makes a successful life, our starting point can't be to study people who are ill or suffering. Instead, we have to start by understanding people who are successful, who are thriving in their lives; the people whom Professor Seligman would describe as flourishing.

This is the study that Maslow undertook. He identified a cohort of people who were flourishing: famous people, people he knew, and even historical figures about whom much was known. And he studied their characteristics and their experiences.

It is worth considering these characteristics and experiences as part of what Maslow considered to be the ultimate life, the ultimate goal to which we all aspire. He described these people as having some or all of these features:

Critical thinking—an astute perception of reality and the ability to reason.

Acceptance of imperfection—accepting and non-judging of themselves and others.

Spontaneous—willing to take risks and experience life to the full.

Higher purpose—they see a problem and feel driven to resolve it, more to the benefit of other people than themselves, 'a task they must do'.

Comfortable with being alone—a strong sense of autonomy and a calmness and confidence in their own abilities. Self-directed.

Fresh appreciation—they seem to be able to always appreciate and express gratitude for their life experiences.

Peak experiences—there is a common description of the moments of high excitement, harmony, and deep meaning, even if they are only momentary.

Connectedness—a strong sense of compassion and caring for others, and a genuine desire to help others.

Humility and respect—treating all people as equal, friendly, and open with all.

Sense of humour—able to laugh at themselves. Non-judgemental in their humour towards others.

Maslow considered specifically the ability of these people to love, including the characteristics of their sex lives, where they were prepared to share them:

The love and sex life of healthy people, in spite of the fact that it frequently reaches great peaks of ecstasy, is nevertheless also easily compared to the games of children and puppies. It is cheerful, humorous, and playful. It is not primarily a striving; it is basically an enjoyment and a delight, which is another thing altogether.[10]

You may or may not agree with the specific characteristics you feel a self-actualized person should have, but this is what Maslow found from his study. A motivation to become the best we can be seems a very worthy goal, however it may be defined, and whatever stage we reach.

What is clear is that these characteristics are not discriminatory in terms of age, gender, race, looks, sexual orientation, ability or disability, relationship, parental status, employment status, or political or religious beliefs.

We can all aspire to be the best we can be, given the resources we have available to us. This is our *why*; this is why the desire to flourish in our lives gives us the motivation to adapt and self-manage in the face of life's challenges. The ability to have health no matter what our circumstances may be.

This is the connection between health and wellbeing, this is the positive health that needs to underpin the new way of medical practice and healthcare.

5

Disability, Chronic Pain, and Medically Unexplained Symptoms

In terms of the new definition of health, the ability to adapt and self-manage in the face of life's challenges, there are few challenges more difficult to face than disability. Nearly a quarter of New Zealanders regard themselves as disabled.

The majority of disabled adults have physical impairments, the commonest (42 per cent) being related to disease or illness. Many of these are disabled because of pain and fatigue, including chronic pain syndromes and chronic fatigue syndrome. Only 22.3 per cent of disabled people were working in 2018, compared to 70 per cent of non-disabled adults.

Hearing and visual impairments are common causes of disability. As much as 10 per cent of disability is due to psychological or psychiatric conditions. In half of disabled children, the disability was present at birth, whether due to congenital conditions, birth trauma, or subsequent developmental issues.

One of my early realizations of the impact of medical practice on people with disabilities occurred a few years ago on a weekend course when I met an inspirational woman called Lucy. I did what doctors often do: they look at people and reach a spot diagnosis. Lucy had a distinctive walk that I thought I recognized. She confirmed she was born with spina bifida—a congenital deformity of the spine that affects the lower end of the spinal cord and causes a degree of paralysis and spasticity in the legs.

I said, 'Yes, I thought that was your disability.'

She immediately corrected me. 'I don't think of it as a disability. I call it my challenge.'

She told me that her hero is Mark Inglis, the man who was the first double amputee to climb Mount Everest. Lucy's aspiration is to trek to Everest Base Camp. Having found out that I was a doctor, she said something that really quite shocked me.

She said, 'I've seen a lot of doctors in my time. Most don't get disability. They don't see me, they only see my spina bifida. Doctors don't see the whole person.'[1]

Positive Medicine. David Beaumont, Oxford University Press. © Oxford University Press 2021.
DOI: 10.1093/oso/9780192845184.003.0006

Many disabled people think they get a raw deal from healthcare. They have difficulty accessing healthcare and when they do, they do not feel their needs are met. The National Centre for Mental Health Research in New Zealand has identified that GPs lack knowledge in the area of disability, with inadequate attention paid to it in their training. They consider that GPs are ill-equipped to respond to the diverse communication needs of disabled people. It would seem as though the healthcare system, and GPs specifically, are not helping people with disability to adapt and self-manage in the face of life's challenges.

In 2015, I had the privilege of delivering the opening keynote presentation to the New Zealand Disability Support Network, an umbrella organization for many different associations who support disabled people. I talked about the relationship between disability, work, and health, and looked at the role played by doctors (including proposing the new way of practice, as a partnership). To prepare, I thought it would be useful to undertake some research specifically aimed at this group, and was introduced to the national executive officer of the New Zealand Down Syndrome Association, Zandra Vaccarino. Zandra's son, Vinnie, is a young adult with Down syndrome, a congenital chromosomal condition which causes multiple disabilities. He also gave a fabulous presentation at the conference.

Zandra readily agreed to undertake some research with me. We did it in two phases. The first phase was a small group discussion with ten young adults with Down syndrome, who form the Strive Group, which advocates for people with Down syndrome. I asked them to consider a series of questions about the care they received from their doctor, and asked them to rate their response on a five-point scale (from 'strongly agree' to 'strongly disagree'). There were nine statements, including:

- Doctors understand my health needs.
- Doctors understand how disability affects my life.
- Doctors treat me with respect.

I was shocked when I received the email from Zandra with the results of the group discussion. For all nine statements, they had given the response, 'strongly disagree'. When I spoke to Zandra, she assured me that this was not the experience of all the group, but when they heard of the problems that some of the group had experienced, the whole group was so incensed that they had agreed to give a wholly negative response. So, we undertook a second phase of the study, to include a group of 100 people of all ages with various different disabilities. The results were considerably more favourable towards doctors than the first phase, with the positive responses ('agree 'or 'strongly agree') to these specific three questions being as follows:

- Doctors understand my health needs—65 per cent.
- Doctors understand how disability affects my life—53 per cent.
- Doctors treat me with respect—77 per cent.

This means that there were still a considerable number of people answering in the negative. Some of their free-text comments were helpful in understanding how these people felt:

It's relative to the doctor you're talking to, which doctor you're seeing. Some are fantastic, some, not so much.

Would be great if doctors had more time, listened and shared all options.

Doctors are totally not tuned in to paediatric special needs. Many are actually scared of me!

As a person with MS [multiple sclerosis] it is common for doctors to misunderstand my condition and needs because MS has no known cause. Doctors that listen and then push to find answers from the medical system are hard to find. The system isn't geared to helping diseases like MS when it focuses on short appointments and throughput of patients.

Many of the negative comments related to system failures, particularly around lack of time. The last comment I've quoted, from a person with multiple sclerosis, really clearly illustrates what I said previously about the medical model. If a diagnosis is reached for which there is no treatment (in a medical sense), then the implication is that the work of the doctor is done, and the residual issues are social problems. One of the comments reflected the sentiment expressed to me by Lucy, my friend with spina bifida: 'For some doctors, all they can see is the disability.'

I want to be really clear, the majority of the comments were positive, and for many, extremely so: 'My doctor is fantastic!' 'The group of doctors who look after our son are great.'

However, it is clear that the experience of some people with disability is that the way the healthcare system is set up does not cater for their needs. Some doctors just don't see the impact of disability on a person's life as being part of the role of the doctor, just as some doctors don't see the fact that someone isn't working as being a factor they need to take into account in their management of a patient.

As a final comment, when I spoke to Zandra recently (and to pass on my congratulations to Vinnie on his recent marriage), she said that recent discussions had focused on the difficulty that some doctors have communicating with people with disabilities when they have a carer present. Often the doctor directs their communication to the carer and not the patient.

Zandra told me that Vinnie has developed a humorous technique for dealing with this whenever it occurs. He says, 'Could you speak to me, please? My mum is just my agent!'

Since 25 per cent of the population consider themselves to be disabled, this is clearly a significant issue. However, it was only when researching disability for the conference, and reading up on some of the concepts by which we understand disability, I came to quite a shocking realization. I learned that, until shortly before the conference, I too had been a disabled person.

Since the majority of disability is caused by illness and disease, it means that any one of us has the potential to develop a disability at some point in our lives. The discussion in Chapter 4 on the concept of health made it clear that health is a dynamic concept; that is, it changes with time and circumstances. So too with disability. With the passage of time, it becomes increasingly likely that we will develop an illness, disease, or injury which impacts the way we function in life to the extent that we meet the definition of disability.

The WHO defines and explains disability in this way:

Disability is an umbrella term, covering impairments, activity limitations, and participation restrictions. An impairment is a problem in bodily function or structure; an activity limitation is a difficulty encountered by an individual in executing a task or action; while a participation restriction is a problem experienced by an individual in involvement in life situations.[2]

My personal story of disability began about 10 years ago, with knee pain. I developed knee pain after an injury, but it didn't resolve and gradually it got worse. An MRI scan showed nothing specific enough to explain it. I saw an orthopaedic surgeon, who examined my knee and again found no specific abnormalities. After examining me more fully, he asked, 'How long have you had hip problems?'

I told him I hadn't had hip problems. He contradicted me and told me that I actually had very limited movement in both hips. Subsequent X-rays identified that I had moderately advanced osteoarthritis in both hips. The pain in my knee had actually been referred pain coming from the hip.

From that time, I had increasing pain and difficulty with activity. Over the next couple of years, movement became more and more painful, until it reached the point that I was in pain constantly, particularly at night (which is a common experience with people with arthritis of various forms). I was avoiding walking up stairs at all cost, had difficulty getting in and out of the car, and could only walk a couple of hundred metres without needing to stop and have a rest, either by sitting down or leaning against a wall.

I recall being in Wellington and going out for a meal with friends. The restaurant was close to the hotel, so we had walked. But when we came out, I was in so much pain that I had to get a taxi to get back. My friends beat me back! By this time, I was on a waiting list for hip replacement surgery, and I was very grateful to the system for having a specific intervention that very effectively removed my pain and gave me back my mobility.

What I hadn't realized until the New Zealand Disability Support Network Conference was that for several years I had experienced at first hand what it means to have a disability—even if only to a slight degree compared to what many people with disability live with on a daily basis.

I learned two other things from this experience. The first happened when I was attending another conference. I was walking through a conference concourse with James Ross, an occupational physician colleague of mine. He asked why I was limping. I explained that I had osteoarthritis in my hips and was awaiting a hip replacement.

I'd seen two orthopaedic surgeons, and both had said the same thing. Even though I was young for a hip replacement (in my early 50s), it was the only course of action given the degree of pain I was in and the lack of effect of painkillers.

James asked me, 'Did they advise you to get active and lose 10 kg?' As I reflected, I realized that they had not. Further, I realized that, even after the warning of having a heart attack, I had still let myself go. I had not been looking after myself properly. My weight had crept up to the point that I had a decent paunch on my belly; and no, I wasn't doing much activity and exercise at all. This was, of course, compounded by the pain from my hips. The reality was that I had settled for the state of being middle-aged—much like the power company's field workers I mentioned in Chapter 4.

With James's question ringing in my ears, I decided that it would be good to get fit before my hip replacement. It was bound to make the recovery quicker. So, I started a nutritional programme to eat more healthily and started a very gradual build-up of exercise.

Gentle walking was good, but even better was aquajogging. This is basically pedalling fast in the water while wearing a floatation belt. This was against the resistance of the water but not weightbearing on my legs, so it was fine for my hips. I found that getting fitter again combined with healthy eating meant that the weight started to drop off me. This meant that I was able to do more, including increasing my walking distance. I had forgotten how much I enjoy walking in nature, and started to look forward to exercise and feel better about myself. My whole mood had lifted. I was in what is called a 'virtuous cycle'. Feeling good about myself and exercise meant I wanted to do more, was more conscientious about my healthy eating, which meant that exercise was easier, which meant I lost more weight.

Suddenly, after 3 months I realized that I had lost 13.5 kg (30 pounds, or over 2 stones). I was walking 10 km several times per week, and here's the kicker—the pain in my hip was much improved! The whole reason for getting fit and active was to prepare for surgery, and I no longer needed surgery! The result was that I put off the surgery for 12 months. I've now had both hips replaced, but the healthy habits I learned from that experience remain with me and my weight and activity levels have improved, along with the benefit of new hips. I feel younger and my family and friends tell me I look younger.

The second thing I learned from this was in relation to the pain itself.

Chronic pain

By the time I was put on a waiting list for hip surgery, my pain had become unbearable. Pain killers made no difference. The pain had changed in character. It was no longer localized to my hip (and the referred pain to my knee). It had spread to my buttocks and down my right leg, all the way to my foot. The pain was no longer sharp and jabbing when I walked, it had become a constant aching, burning, throbbing pain.

I just couldn't get comfortable, no matter what position I got into. In bed at night was the worst. I took to sleeping with a pillow between my legs, but even then, my sleep was dreadfully disturbed, and I often got up in the night. I started having massages on my buttocks, because the muscles themselves had become really tender, with tender trigger points.

It was only 2 years after the hip replacement, listening to a lecture at a pain conference, that I realized what had happened. I had developed a chronic pain syndrome.

You will have gathered by now that I regard definitions of words as extremely important if we are to truly understand their implications. I have found that 'chronic pain' is a term that often causes a fear reaction in patients.

There are two reasons for this. First, the diagnosis is often accompanied by the doctor telling the patient that they are difficult to treat. The second is that the word 'chronic' is often misunderstood.

I once saw a young woman for a rehabilitation programme who had just been given the diagnosis of a chronic pain syndrome. She told me that she had not heard of it previously, but was scared as to the implications. When I asked her why she felt scared, she explained, 'Well, it's chronic. You know, really bad.'

As a medical term, chronic does not mean really bad; it simply means persistent or long term. A chronic illness is not necessarily a bad one, but it is one that has been long-lasting. In pain specifically, it means has lasted more than 3 months. It often brings considerable relief to explain that this is all that the word means, and that there are techniques to learn to be able to manage the pain.

A chronic pain syndrome often means that the pain has continued longer than would be expected for the degree of the injury, or long after healing or recovery would have been expected, or is considerably worse than would be expected for the degree of tissue damage. Such pain may even occur in the absence of any damage to the tissue.

What I heard at the pain conference was that chronic pain syndromes are common in patients with osteoarthritis of the hip and knee, and that this is often not recognized by doctors, particularly the orthopaedic surgeons who perform the joint replacements.

As I listened to the description of the widening of the area of pain, the hypersensitivity to touch, and the presence of allodynia (when normal touch or temperature changes at the skin feel unpleasantly painful), a dreadful burning, aching sensation, I realized that I had been experiencing a chronic pain syndrome, which had never been diagnosed, including by myself!

More importantly, the presenter explained the mechanism by which chronic pain syndromes are now understood. It is a process occurring in the brain known as central sensitization.

Of the thousands of people I have seen who have not gone back to work after a prolonged period of time, many have had pain, many have had chronic pain syndromes, and therefore they have been experiencing the phenomenon of central sensitization.

I want to explain it carefully, because it is an essential component to understanding the interaction between the brain and the musculoskeletal system and organs. The link between mind and body. It is an important concept, well known and understood by pain specialist doctors. But from my experience, it is either not known or not understood by the many doctors who are *not* specializing in pain. This lack of knowledge is, in my opinion, a root cause of iatrogenesis, namely the inadvertent harm caused by doctors.

Central sensitization was first described in 1983 by Clifford Woolf, a professor of neurology and neurobiology at Harvard Medical School. He described the concept that, although pain can arise from tissue damage or pathology and direct stimulation of peripheral nerves, it can also occur as a result of hypersensitivity to pain itself. This occurs because of mechanisms in the central nervous system (primarily the brain), even in the absence of any tissue damage. Over the years since, Woolf has contributed massively to our understanding of this pain phenomenon through research and publication. His explanation has been confirmed through such investigations as functional MRI scans, which demonstrate changes in the function of the brain in such conditions, and is widely accepted.

To understand the concept properly, it is necessary to go back in time to the evolution of our human species. I have already mentioned the concept of homeostasis—the ability of the body to maintain its functions within finely tuned limits (body temperature, blood pressure, blood chemistry, etc.). In order to achieve this fine balance, we have evolved incredibly complex feedback mechanisms. They detect changes in our environment and within ourselves and bring into play bodily systems to correct these changes and keep our systems in a state of balance.

One of the things that challenges the body to respond with a homeostatic mechanism is the threat of danger, particularly the threat of damage to tissues. We react in various ways to such danger, bringing into play the flight or fight response, involving the nervous system, the hormonal system, and the immune system. This prepares the muscles for the action they need to take, activates the sympathetic nervous system to increase heart rate and release adrenaline and inflammatory substances into the bloodstream in preparation for repair of tissue damage. If tissue damage occurs, or there is perception of damage to tissues, then all of these functions are increased by the brain's perception of pain. Pain is a state of fear in response to a threat of tissue damage. The definition of pain used by the International Association for the Study of Pain is 'an unpleasant sensory and emotional experience associated with actual or potential tissue damage, or described in terms of such damage'.[3]

I understand central sensitization best as an escalation of this primitive defence mechanism from the presence of a pain cycle. If pain is generated from the tissues and interpreted as pain by the brain, then the mechanisms to correct this, to restore homeostasis, are activated. We withdraw or flee from the stimulus. If tissues have been damaged, then we start the process of healing with the intention that the pain subsides. In central sensitization, the brain mechanisms are overstimulated and become oversensitive, overprotective of the body, and the pain does not subside.[4]

The following are the cases of four people I have seen to provide advice to on rehabilitation:

John was referred to me because he had been off work for 4 months with a diagnosis of carpal tunnel syndrome. But his case was atypical. He had the sensory changes and tingling in his right hand, and he had pain, which is common in this condition. However, the gold standard test for the condition, known as nerve conduction studies, were entirely normal. In addition, the distribution of the neurological symptoms wasn't typical, and the pain was far more widespread and severe. I examined him and found that not only were the classical tests for carpal tunnel syndrome (Tinel's test and Phalen's test) negative, but I actually couldn't find any physical abnormality. In short, the diagnosis he had been given, by both his GP and orthopaedic surgeon who wanted to operate on the 'trapped nerve' he didn't have, was incorrect. (The diagnosis is incorrect in a significant proportion of the cases I see.)

Because I specialize in the health of workers, it is important for me to understand the job that a person does, and the specific functions of that job, so I enquire in detail. John had an interesting job: he was a turkey inseminator. As I often find in my consultations, John himself gave me the answer and the diagnosis.

He said to me, 'My job involves inseminating a thousand turkeys a day, weighing up to 20 kg [44 pounds]. I grab them round the legs with my right hand, swing them up and over so they're upside down, and then inseminate them with a syringe in my left hand. In the first few weeks I got his awful aching and burning in my right forearm. I spoke to the other guys and they said, "That always happens to start with. You'll get used to it and it will go away." But it didn't; it got worse.'

Employers encourage their workers to report pain and discomfort early, so that it can be managed and not develop into what John had.

Because the cycle of pain had persisted, it had become entrenched into sensory centres in the brain which process pain. John had developed a hyperarousal state in these centres, so that he had a central sensitization—a condition called a regional pain syndrome. When it occurs in the arms in this way it used to be called repetitive strain injury, or RSI. This term has now largely gone out of usage, because there is no injury as such to the tissues. Instead, the disorder is a reflection of a dysfunction in the processing of nerve signals from the periphery by the brain.

I had not found any abnormality when examining John's arm, in fact, not even tenderness in the muscles. And yet, every time he tried to go back to work the pain was so severe, he couldn't even last a day. He explained, 'Even picking up the landline phone is painful.'

As he said this, he mimicked the action of reaching down to a telephone and lifting it to his ear. As he did so, he gasped with pain. 'Ow! That's it—that's the pain!'

Reaching down to the phone and lifting it up involved the same muscles doing the same movements as when he lifted a turkey. The fact that the phone weighed next to nothing in comparison to a turkey didn't matter to his brain. His brain was in overprotective and overdefensive mode. This is a hypersensitivity state. John's brain was screaming at him to stop doing that activity for fear of tissue damage.

I worked with him and his employer to put together a multidisciplinary rehabilitation programme (involving a physiotherapist, occupational therapist, psychologist, and myself). We soon had him back at work and pain free.

Brian was a greater challenge. He had not worked for 3 years when I saw him. He had developed carpal tunnel syndrome and had had surgical release of the trapped nerve in his wrist, but had developed a regional pain syndrome after the surgery.

Chronic pain after surgery is a common occurrence. It is a reason why surgery in painful conditions has to be considered carefully, and why pre- and postoperative pain relief is so important. My experience of the way that multidisciplinary pain management has developed in New Zealand leads me to believe it is the closest way of practising to the new way of medical practice that I view as the way forward for medicine.

Many occupational physicians include pain management in their practice because of the holistic view of health and functionality that they hold. Returning to work and full participation in life's activities are very much seen as part of treatment. The role of occupational physicians and pain specialists is often to reduce or stop medication (particularly opiates like morphine and codeine), rather than initiating treatment. Pain management is based on an empowerment model: helping people to understand their condition and their pain, and to self-manage rather than rely on treatment, or the 'fix' that usually isn't there. We help them develop an 'internal locus of control': a belief in their own ability to manage their pain and to get on with their lives despite pain, in the hope and expectation that the pain will diminish.

We developed a multidisciplinary team to work with Brian. It comprised a physiotherapist to help him with exercise to build up the use of the muscles in his arms and get the brain used to the arm functioning more normally, and also to help him improve his general fitness (he had become unfit and deconditioned while off work for 3 years); an occupational therapist to help him to structure his day and incorporate the exercise programme, and also to help him get a better sleep pattern; and a psychologist to help him understand his pain better, and help him to see the advantages for himself and his family if he could take control of his own situation, to help him understand that he needed to work through the pain to achieve the rewards of moving forward with his life. As a team, we met with Brian and his employer, who, even after 3 years, was keen to support Brian to return to work.

I phoned his specialist to talk about the planned return to work. I met a degree of resistance which still shocks me to this day: 'No. Absolutely not. He's in pain. I've got a list of 15 drugs I'm trialling. We've tried 12 so far, and no combination has helped him. He is not to return to work until we've exhausted the medication possibilities.'

I've got to call it out—this is iatrogenesis: inadvertent harm caused by doctors.

It's also reflective of the old way, the way that says, 'There are symptoms, we've only got to get the medication right'; the way that says that someone has to be 100 per cent fit to return to work.

The evidence and modern practice both show that we don't get better to go back to work, we go back to work to get better. Professor Clifford Woolf says that doctors' treatment of pain has not improved in the last 20 years; that the empirical way of trial and error in pain treatment needs to be replaced by an approach that reflects the underlying mechanisms that we now recognize to exist in chronic pain.

Sadly, patients' own expectations are set by their doctors. People expect to be prescribed medication for pain, but all the evidence is that modern medication for pain is not particularly effective. This leads to false expectations, and the erroneous view that it is only a matter of trying different drugs to find the one that works.

We had a fantastic breakthrough with Brian. He was starting to understand his pain better, starting to re-engage with his hobbies and his friends. At one of his review meetings with me he was very excited to tell me a story. He said, 'I've just been with the family to Christchurch for the weekend. My mate took me to the pub on Saturday evening, and there was a poker tournament. I love playing poker! Guess what? I won the tournament! $800! But this is the big one—I woke the next morning and I was still buzzing from the night. I suddenly realized I had no pain in my arm. None! And what's more, I couldn't remember having had any pain while I was playing poker.' His pain had returned by the time I saw him, but he had hope, for the first time in 3 years. He had heard the team reassuring him that he could take control of his own pain, and here was the experience that gave him evidence this could be the case.

Intuitively, we know that pain is worse when we're upset or angry. The converse is also true. When we're in a state of extreme emotion such as happiness or excitement, then pain is diminished. Pain is an emotional response, and so it can be modified.

It's hard not to be in a state of fear or anger when you're going through chronic pain. Many of the people I have seen over the years have been angry. One of the things they get angry about is when a doctor or health professional tries to explain their pain. I have had many patients say, angrily, 'You're trying to tell me it's all in my head!', particularly when the concept of having them see a psychologist is suggested.

I've learnt techniques over the years to pre-empt this response, and even turn it round to advantage. It's never worked better than when I saw *Neil*, a tough farmer with low back pain who hadn't worked for 2 years. Central sensitization and chronic pain are common accompaniments to low back pain. I asked Neil to consider what happens when you step on a drawing pin: where do you feel the pain?

As is always the response, he said (somewhat grumpily), 'In your foot, of course.'

I immediately countered by saying, 'No, you don't; you feel it in your brain. All of our senses are interpreted in our brain. A signal is sent from sensors in the skin of the foot as a nerve impulse to the brain, where the brain interprets the sensation as noxious and we react. In fact, there is a reflex that occurs at a spinal level that causes the leg muscles to contract and move your foot so fast that your foot moves before you even experience pain.'

He looked at me blankly for a minute. I must admit to a degree of apprehension as to how he was going to respond. Then he burst out laughing. 'Oh my goodness, for all this time I've been getting angry when I thought people were suggesting it's all in my head, and it *is* all in my head!'

From that point we were able to have a really constructive conversation regarding the interaction between what was going on in his back and how his brain was interpreting the signals. I explained central sensitization to him in a way he could relate to, and that empowered him to understand the programme we were designing for him.

Another way I seek to empower patients is in discussing their pain medication with them. *Belinda* was angry and grumpy. I had been warned that she was fed up with the attempts that kept being made to control her pain and were getting nowhere. She had been referred for me to review her pain medication.

I said to her, 'There's an expert in pain medication in this room … and it isn't me.'

'What do you mean? I thought you were meant to be an expert? Are you wasting my time?'

'Not at all', I said. 'But there's no one in the world who knows your pain as well as you do, and no one who knows better what works and what doesn't.'

Belinda said, 'Well, gabapentin doesn't work, I'll tell you that!'

Pain is, by definition, subjective. It's an experience that happens in our brain, it can't be measured, and no one knows what we're experiencing but us. Pain medication is also very individual in terms of what works and what doesn't.

Gabapentin (Neurontin®) can be very effective, but it has unpleasant side effects and patients often don't like taking it. An important fact that comes from the research evidence about gabapentin is that NNT, or number needed to treat, is between 6 and 8. The NNT is a way of evaluating the effectiveness of drugs. What it means in this case is that between six and eight people need to be treated with gabapentin in order to find one person who benefits, with a 50 per cent reduction in pain. Yes, it should be trialled; but if it isn't effective, it should be stopped.

People with chronic pain often finish up on cocktails of drugs and therefore they experience the risk of side effects unnecessarily. On the other hand, Belinda said that paracetamol was as effective as anything that was prescribed for her. I asked how many she was taking. The answer was two tablets, two or three times per week.

Because paracetamol isn't prescribed, it often isn't taken regularly even when patients find it effective. We completely revamped Belinda's regimen—but I only facilitated and validated the process by listening to what she had to say. I helped her realize that she truly was the expert in her own condition and its management.

Medically unexplained symptoms

Chronic pain caused by central sensitization is a medically unexplained symptom. That is, it's medically unexplained by the medical model. Chronic pain is present in many different conditions. It can affect any and every part of the body. The examination findings of a doctor are often either negative or non-specific and hard to explain. Investigations in the form of blood tests and

X-rays are usually normal. No cause can be found, no specific pathology identified. But reading the research papers by Professor Woolf and many other eminent pain specialists, chronic pain has a very clear underlying mechanism and explanation.

What are 'medically unexplained symptoms'? The term covers a large group of conditions which often have vague descriptive names and for which there is no consensus about their underlying cause. Often, they are painful conditions and can be causes of chronic pain. Frequently, they are associated with a feeling of fatigue. They are also associated with disorders of function of some part of the body or organ system. Common examples include fibromyalgia, chronic fatigue syndrome (also known as ME, myalgic encephalomyelitis, or ME/CFS), irritable bowel syndrome, irritable bladder syndrome, non-cardiac chest pain, and unexplained pelvic pain. Even common conditions such as headache and depression are 'medically unexplained'.

Because no consensus has been reached and they remain officially unexplained, we don't know the cause (the aetiology) of these conditions. As we don't know the cause, it can be argued there *is* no specific treatment or cure. Because we don't have a specific treatment, then maybe there's nothing doctors can do, and therefore the prognosis (the likelihood of recovery) remains uncertain, and probably poor. But worse than this bleak (some would say cynical) view of the situation, it means that patients who suffer from these conditions can be left with the feeling that doctors believe that it's all in their heads.

As I listen to the debate, I hear three schools of thought regarding what these conditions are:

- They are diseases for which we have not yet identified the underlying pathology, and for which more research is needed.
- They are in some way psychological conditions, with thought processes resulting in generation of symptoms.
- They are disorders of function of the interaction between the brain and the organs and/or the musculoskeletal system.

The problem with such diverse opinions and lack of definitive agreement is that it pushes people into camps, and creates strength of opinion and increases the likelihood of someone adopting the position of 'we're right, therefore you're wrong'. It can mean that, when research does identify possible explanations, efforts are put into criticizing or discrediting the conclusions. Why can't we just put all of the findings into the mix, not become fixed on one explanation, and keep our minds open to the possibility that the true answer lies in a combination of 'all of the above'?

Why *can't* we do that? Why does it have to be so black or white?

I believe one reason is explained by the concept of 'Cartesian dualism'. Named after the seventeenth-century philosopher René Descartes, it was the concept that the mind and the body are two separate things. Two parts of the whole, perhaps, but the body is physical and mechanistic and the mind, and consciousness, ethereal and even mystical. The body was seen to be the domain of doctors, and the mind of the Church. Current criticism of the medical model includes the observation that it focuses on the physical, tangible, and measurable, and does not take into account the mind and the effect that life and life experience has on the functioning of the whole. This flies in the face of our increasing understanding of the science of human functioning: our thoughts affect our bodies, and the experience of our bodies affects our thought processes. Further, who we are, our genetic makeup, which makes us unique, is far from set in stone. The science of epigenetics has clearly demonstrated that who we are and who we will become are very much affected by our environment and our life experiences. How our genes are expressed is shaped by our life, positive or negative.

What if the true answer is a combination of all of these explanations?

Professor Clifford Woolf thinks it is. He identifies evidence of central sensitization in many of these conditions, raising the possibility of a common underlying mechanism, with a dysfunctional relationship between the central and autonomic nervous system and the immune system. The new science of neuroimmunology is identifying the extent to which the nervous system and the immune system are intimately interrelated. They are not separate, but integral to the whole. It is the attempt by the system to find homeostasis, to return the organism to balance, that causes the dysfunction. In producing dysfunction, the organs do not function properly, the nervous system is hypersensitive and overly defensive, and the immune system attacks an invisible and fictional enemy, releasing inflammatory chemicals in the process. All this results in chronic pain, chronic fatigue, and dysfunctional organ processes.

Granted, in many of these conditions, abnormalities have been identified in the immune system along with raised inflammatory markers, though not sufficient to identify them as distinct inflammatory conditions. Yes, that *does* indicate the need for more research. However, the finding of such abnormalities does not indicate whether they provide evidence of an underlying disorder causing illness, or whether they are in themselves the product of system dysfunction.

Curing versus healing

There is much overlap in the symptoms of these conditions, meaning that even symptom combinations can't be used to identify them as truly separate syndromes. More than this, they often coexist, so patients with ME/CFS often have widespread pain similar to fibromyalgia and may also have irritable bowel syndrome and chronic headaches. Most importantly of all, these conditions are common, accounting for between a third and half of all GP consultations and attendances in hospital outpatient clinics. That is a massive reason to get this right.

What if we acknowledge that, regardless of exactly *what* these conditions are, they are real conditions that cause very real disability?

What if the answer to what is required is to assist the organism to achieve homeostasis, to find balance?

Saying, 'We don't know what they are so we don't have a treatment' doesn't allow for the fact that there is sound evidence for the effectiveness of two, maybe three modalities of management that apply to many of these conditions: graded exercise therapy, cognitive behavioural therapy, and where depression coexists, perhaps antidepressants (although the evidence for antidepressants is weakest).

What if to achieve homeostasis and balance we need to truly hear people who suffer from the effects of these conditions and help empower them to adapt and self-manage so they can live their lives to the full? Return to life, return to health. My son, Matt, taught me that this is the new way that medical students in New Zealand are being taught. If doctors can't cure, then their role is to help patients heal—to learn to manage their symptoms and adapt their lives to live them to the full.

Cole's Medical Practice in New Zealand is the guide to the practice of medicine that all New Zealand doctors are encouraged to refer to. It acknowledges that in relation to the concept of patient-centred clinical medicine, 'most senior doctors have not been explicitly trained in its use'. It explains further the concept of curing versus healing:

> The goal with the former is cure, or at least modification of the disease process. The goal with the latter is modification of the illness experience through relief of suffering, professional guidance, support and long-term care. The goal of this interpersonal relationship is to help the patient gain greater tolerance and equanimity in the face of disease.[5]

In contrast to this description is the effect of medical care on a 57-year-old woman I saw together with her husband. Her insurance company had asked me to review her on the tenth anniversary of her claim on her income protection policy to confirm whether or not she was still disabled from work. She had a diagnosis of chronic fatigue syndrome (ME/CFS). At the time I saw her, she was in bed for 22 hours of the day, apart from 2 hours in the evening, when her husband would help her out of bed to have dinner and watch a little television. He had given up work years ago in order to care for her. Quality of life? Very low, for both of them. Ability to return to work? Zero.

I asked what management she had received from her GP. They both looked confused.

'He said there isn't any treatment.'

I was left with a feeling of profound sadness. The risk of the medical model is this: if there is no known cause, there is no treatment, therefore nothing further needs to occur. That's not enabling healing, that's iatrogenesis—inadvertent harm caused by doctors.

There are signs of change. Gastroenterologists are now more likely to refer to irritable bowel syndrome as 'functional gastrointestinal disorder'. There is wider recognition of the connection in this condition of a disorder of function between the bowel and its connections with the autonomic nervous system and the associated central sensitization.

In June 2018, the WHO announced its 11th revision of the International Classification of Disease (ICD-11). Ratified by the World Health Assembly in May 2019, and coming into effect in January 2022, it brings together for the first time the various medically unexplained symptoms under one diagnostic label, that of bodily distress disorder.[6] Although the new term has been criticized by some, particularly those who believe that there is sufficient evidence for ME/CFS to have its own diagnostic label and therefore be considered separately, I see this new term as acknowledging the suffering caused by these conditions and opening the way for more research into both causation and management aimed at cure or, at least, healing.

6

Why Should Health and Wellbeing Matter to Doctors?

When I told a doctor friend, a published author, that I was writing a book that brings medicine and health and wellbeing together, he said, 'Sounds too much like a personal development book. Doctors won't read it.'

I think he was wrong. At least, I think he was partly wrong. Some won't read it, and that's OK. But some will welcome it. It's those doctors that I'm reaching out to—which means you, if you're a doctor who has read this far. And if the $4 trillion spent globally each year on health and wellbeing is anything to go by, patients are looking for a more whole-person and holistic approach to health.

The concept of health and wellbeing as part of medical practice should matter to doctors. It's what many of their patients are looking for in their lives. (As a non-fiction genre, health and wellbeing is one of the most popular topics.) It should matter because we're losing the battle against the epidemic of the diseases of lifestyle in the Western world. We need to move into the prevention of disease, not merely mitigating harm once it has occurred. In fact, increasingly I'm realizing that we need to go even further beyond prevention of disease, to the enhancement of health.

The other side of the equation is that doctors should be concerned for their own health and wellbeing, and their patients should too. Unhealthy doctors provide poorer care to their patients.

How doctors can change the world

In 2015/2016, I was president of the Australasian Faculty of Occupational and Environmental Medicine (AFOEM), the professional body of all specialist occupational physicians in Australia and New Zealand. The Faculty is part of the Royal Australasian College of Physicians (RACP), which is the training, education, and advocacy body for all specialist physicians and paediatricians in Australian and New Zealand—all 25,000 specialists and specialist doctors in

Positive Medicine. David Beaumont, Oxford University Press. © Oxford University Press 2021.
DOI: 10.1093/oso/9780192845184.003.0007

training. It meant I was a director on the Board of the College at a time when the Board had a problem with the annual conference of the College, known as Congress. Our doctors were not attending it because they saw it as staid and traditional. Congress was essentially a series of lectures on scientific, medical subjects. Clearly our members wanted something different.

A Congress Lead Fellow, Dr Michael Gabbett, was appointed to change the Congress model. A 'shared interest' model was developed. Michael chaired the committee to define the programme. What subjects would be of interest to cardiologists, respiratory physicians, paediatricians, public health physicians, and the myriad of other specialties represented by the College? It turned out to be cutting-edge topics by leading international experts, topics where the role of doctors is in transition, where doctors need to consider carefully what their role is; areas like medicinal marijuana, physician-assisted dying, the care of asylum seekers, and climate change.

Ultimately, the shared interest model received 95 per cent satisfaction ratings from Congress delegates. It was agreed that the direction was correct, and that we needed to be braver, to disrupt the model of Congress further, to really push the thinking of doctors so that participation at the Congress would be a challenging and active process, and not a passive soaking up of information.

Sir Harry Burns gave the closing plenary address at that first Congress. Sir Harry is Professor of Global Health in Glasgow, and was formerly the Chief Medical Officer for Scotland. It was Sir Harry's talk that made me want to take on the role of Congress Lead Fellow after Michael.

Sir Harry challenged the audience to consider how doctors can change the world. The answer, he said, lay not in getting better at being experts in disease management, but in truly understanding what makes people ill or healthy; changing our role, and our practice, to prevent ill health and improve health and wellbeing. The answer lay in the social determinants of health, particularly early childhood experiences.

Sir Harry introduced us to the work of Aaron Antonovsky who, in his 1979 book *Health, Stress, and Coping*, proposed that we could understand the association between health and disease as a continuum, that at any one time we all have different degrees of both health and disease.[1] It's a balance. Antonovsky saw the link between the two as being stress, and particularly our ability to cope with stress, or more specifically, with stressors. Stressors are the events, experiences, environment, and challenges that we all face in life. The extent to which we experience stressors, and the way that we respond to them, determines where we sit on the continuum he described as having 'ease' at one end, and 'dis-ease' at the other.

Antonovsky thought the medical establishment was getting it wrong in the way it approached the understanding of the basis of development of disease (pathogenesis). The approach was to start with a condition such as cardiovascular disease, or cancer, and undertake research to understand the condition. But Antonovsky thought that, at the 'dis-ease' end of the spectrum, the state of 'dis-ease' may or may not cause disease; and that if it did, it could be one of many different kinds. The body has many different mechanisms to remain in a state of function and balance (the process of homeostasis). In stress states, the mechanisms to return the body to normal function and balance become overwhelmed. Antonovsky proposed that the difference in where we are on the continuum of health ease or dis-ease depended on our belief in our ability to use our resources to deal with the stressors of life. Our belief in our ability to control our own destiny; that is, having an internal locus of control.

Sir Harry showed us a very clear association between chronic stress and disease, particularly stress in childhood, and the later development of adult diseases. When a child is exposed to physical, sexual, or emotional abuse, or neglect, or domestic violence, they run a greater risk of adult diseases of all kinds, depending on the degree of adversity they have experienced in childhood.

Much of our understanding of the relationship between adverse childhood experiences (ACEs) and adult ill health and poor social outcomes comes from the Adverse Childhood Experiences Study in the US. This collaboration between health maintenance organization Kaiser Permanente and the Centres for Disease Control and Prevention recruited over 17,000 volunteers between 1995 and 1997, and has been measuring their health and social outcomes in relation to ACEs, producing many scientific studies. The inaugural study identified a strong graded relationship between the number of ACEs and the leading causes of adult morbidity and mortality.[2]

If we all face stressors, why don't we all get stressed?

Well, of course, the answer is that we all do, at some point or other. What differentiates us is the extent and duration of that stress. In the face of an acute stressor, our mechanisms are there to protect us. Our sympathetic nervous system releases adrenaline to prepare us for flight or fight. But before that level of defence is provoked, we assess whether we have the resources to cope with challenges, and if we believe we do, then we step up and improve our performance. The human performance curve shows how with increasing levels of challenge our performance improves.

A degree of challenge and exposure to stressors is healthy. The opposite of 'stress' is called *eustress*, healthy stress, if you like. But at a certain point, our system becomes overwhelmed and our performance crashes: we become stressed. That point varies from person to person, according to our belief in our ability to cope. At that point, with more sustained stress, the body has a second mechanism to protect us and return us to balance, or homeostasis. This mechanism begins in the brain. Inputs from the environment are received by the tiny region of the brain known as the amygdala, the primitive fear centre of the body. Triggering the amygdala does two things. First, it causes us to evaluate the degree of threat, by sending signals to our higher centres in the more evolutionary advanced cortex of the brain, and specifically the area behind the forehead, the prefrontal cortex. This is where we seek to understand and rationalize our world. If we can explain the threat in terms we can understand and manage, and bring our resources into play, then the fear response can be damped down.

If not, a cascade of events starts to occur that prepares the body to deal with the consequences of the threat. The amygdala triggers the hypothalamus–pituitary–adrenal (HPA) axis. The HPA axis begins in the brain, with the hypothalamus releasing a hormone (corticotrophin-releasing hormone, CRH) which causes the pituitary to release a hormone (adrenocorticotrophic hormone, ACTH), which triggers the adrenal glands (which sit on top of the kidneys) to release steroid hormones (glucocorticoids), including cortisol (Fig. 6.1). This is the connection between the nervous system and the immune system in stress. The release of these steroid hormones acts as a potent anti-inflammatory agent. Many chronic diseases are associated with chronic inflammation, so a response to stress that aims to revert the body to balance by producing anti-inflammatory substances does not in itself seem to provide evidence of a link between stress and chronic disease.

The process by which the brain responds to stressors and attempts to respond to the threat and return the body to balance (homeostasis) is termed *allostasis*. In our evolutionary history, we were more likely to behave in the same way as animals respond to the threat of a predator. If we were threatened by a sabre-toothed tiger, then our flight or fight and stress responses would kick in. Once the danger had passed, the process of allostasis would return the body to its normal state of ease.

Modern life isn't like that. Even after acute events, we remain to some degree under the influence of stressors (particularly if our system has been programmed by childhood trauma to be in a state of fear). That residual stress effect is called allostatic load. It's this residual effect on the brain, sympathetic nervous system, and HPA axis that results in dysfunction of the normal

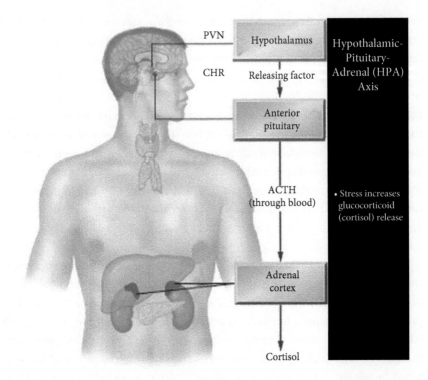

Fig. 6.1 The hypothalamus–pituitary–adrenal axis and the stress response.

process. Sir Harry showed us MRI scans of the brain in chronic stress. In the presence of allostatic load, there are measurable structural changes in the brain. The fear centre—the amygdala—enlarges, and the prefrontal cortex shrinks. The brain becomes more sensitive to fear and less able to reason and respond using its higher, cortical cognitive functions. All this is visible on an MRI scan.

If homeostasis is the function of keeping the body's systems within a certain range of preset limits, then allostasis allows the body to reset those limits in response to perceived ongoing stress. It is the resetting of these limits to a perception of threat that causes a chronic state of dis-ease. The pressure of modern life, primed by childhood experiences, all adds to this allostatic load.

It is only in recent years that our understanding has grown as to how the anti-inflammatory effects of cortisol production in normal states relate to the impact of the allostatic load in dysfunctional states of chronic stress, and therefore may link to disease production. The evidence comes from the work of a number of researchers, but a very elegant piece of research was conducted by Professor Sheldon Cohen. Professor Cohen and his team undertook a series of experiments on healthy volunteers and assessed them for the degree of stress in their lives and then deliberately exposed them to the cold virus (rhinovirus). They found that people under stress are more prone to develop infection and get a cold.

Next, they took the concept further and researched the immune system to find what was happening. They found that people under stress are less able to regulate the inflammatory response, and when exposed to the cold virus they are more likely to release inflammatory chemicals (pro-inflammatory cytokines) and develop a cold. Although they found cortisol to be elevated in chronic stress, the body becomes less responsive to its effects, and paradoxically develops an inflammatory state. They termed this 'glucocorticoid receptor resistance'.

In an interview, Professor Cohen explained:

The immune system's ability to regulate inflammation predicts who will develop a cold, but more importantly it provides an explanation of how stress can promote disease.

When under stress, cells of the immune system are unable to respond to hormonal control, and consequently, produce levels of inflammation that promote disease. Because inflammation plays a role in many diseases such as cardiovascular, asthma and autoimmune disorders, this model suggests why stress impacts them as well.[3]

This is an entirely plausible explanation, because an analogous response occurs with a different hormone, in diabetes. Insulin is the body's hormone that regulates homeostasis of blood glucose and keeps it within a finely tuned band of normality. In type 1 diabetes, there is a deficiency of insulin which causes blood glucose to rise uncontrollably, requiring insulin to be administered artificially by injection. But the modern epidemic of diabetes is due to type 2 diabetes, the form commonly associated with being overweight and often sedentary. In this form, the levels of insulin are chronically high, but the tissues that normally respond to insulin to remove glucose from the bloodstream become insensitive to the stimulus from insulin—they become insulin resistant. What is more, there is increasing evidence that chronic inflammatory states are also part of the underlying mechanism for developing diabetes. It is this insulin resistance that is the underlying mechanism for the collection of abnormalities known as metabolic syndrome, which includes raised blood sugar, hypertension, raised cholesterol, and increased body fat around the waist. It leads to increased risk of heart disease and stroke.

Professor Cohen points out that, despite growing evidence for the role of stress in the development of disease, 'the biomedical community remains sceptical of this conclusion'. Despite this scepticism among some doctors, increasingly the view is developing that inflammation is the common pathway in the development of stress-related diseases.

Here we have scientific evidence to support Antonovsky's model of health being a continuum between ease and dis-ease, that the state of dis-ease is a condition of chronic stress associated with low-grade chronic inflammation, which is pathogenic, that is, it can cause disease. So, you can be in a state of chronic stress and dis-ease, but not have disease. But perhaps the disease is just waiting to happen, and if you do get a disease it could be type 2 diabetes, or cancer, or cardiovascular disease, or Alzheimer's disease—all diseases that have been demonstrated to be associated with chronic inflammation.

Here's an interesting twist. The medically unexplained symptoms—low-grade inflammation and immune system abnormalities—that have been identified in conditions such as chronic fatigue syndrome are also associated with chronic inflammation. There is also a clear association between adverse childhood events (including serious physical, emotional, and sexual abuse) and the development of these conditions. What if sufferers from medically unexplained symptoms are in a state of dis-ease, just as those who get diabetes or cancer? Surely they deserve the same degree of medical care as sufferers of these more manifestly 'physical' conditions?

Sir Harry introduced us to the concept of perceived control (remember, this was a 40-minute lecture—the ground-breaking concepts covered in that time were mind-blowing to the audience). He told us that Antonovsky had pointed out that if the model of health as a continuum between ease and dis-ease was correct, then we can use it for promotion of health. We can help people shift from the dis-ease end of the spectrum towards the ease end. He suggested three requirements to achieve this. Firstly, we have to be able to comprehend and understand the challenges that we encounter in life, from within ourselves and our environment, and make sense of them (the function of our prefrontal cortex). Secondly, we need to have the belief that we have the resources, or can find the resources, to manage our challenges (perceived control); and finally, we have to feel that life is meaningful—in other words, that living our lives in a meaningful way makes it worth the effort to take control of our circumstances.

Sir Harry showed us the international research that demonstrates these relationships very clearly. The lower our belief in the perceived control of our lives, the greater is our all-cause mortality. This is known as our *locus of control*. If we believe we control our own destinies, we have an internal locus of control; if we believe that what happens in our lives is outside our control, we are said to have an external locus of control. The feeling you experience if you have an external locus of control in the face of life's challenges is hopelessness.

The figures Sir Harry showed us were astounding. If you are a person with a high sense of hopelessness in the face of life's challenges, you have a risk of death from all causes that is three-and-a-half times greater than someone with an internal locus of control. Similar figures apply to cardiovascular disease and cancer. Here we come right back to the new definition of health.

Health is the ability to adapt and self-manage in the face of life's challenges. Health is the ability to develop an internal locus of control!

One last concept Sir Harry introduced into the mix came from the new science of epigenetics. Since the 1990s, a large body of research has shown that how our genetic make-up is expressed, including our propensity to the development of disease, is influenced by effects on our DNA from environmental factors, that is, factors outside ourselves. They include lifestyle factors such as diet, inactivity, and smoking—and also stress. Changes in glucocorticosteroid receptors (the receptors for cortisol) have been found in adults who were exposed to adverse childhood events. These changes may increase their likelihood of developing disease, and because the changes affect DNA they are passed from cell to cell, including being heritable by the next generation.

Doctors must do more to change the world

Sir Harry Burns's closing oration at Congress 2016 was a massive turning point for me as a doctor. A number of colleagues who were there felt the same. This was the validation I needed, that there is a new way. I felt that, despite the scepticism of traditional medicine, there is a clear scientific evidence base that seeing health and disease as a dichotomy (an either/or) is simplistic, reductionist, and—from where I sit now, reviewing the evidence—completely wrong. That the role of doctors, and therefore the practice of medicine, has to evolve with our changing understanding of what health truly is. That we have to shift to the preventative side of the equation and, dare I say it, embrace some of the concepts purveyed by the health and wellbeing sector.

In 2017, I was asked to chair the closing plenary of the annual RACP Congress. The session was to follow the theme of Sir Harry Burns's talk, 'How doctors can change the world', and was provocatively titled 'Doctors must do more to change the world'.

The world's authority on the association between our life circumstances and our health is probably Sir Michael Marmot. I asked Sir Michael to be part of the session. He was the chair of the WHO's Commission on the Social Determinants of Health. He is a public health physician who famously investigated the health of Britain's civil service in the Whitehall studies (known as Whitehall I and II).

The Whitehall I study began in 1967. For 10 years, the health of 17,500 male civil servants was monitored, with a particular focus on cardiovascular disease. The civil service had a quintessentially British organizational hierarchy: tier after tier of management and layers of seniority and status. What did they find? Intuitively, we may reason that the higher up the organization, the more the pressure, the more likely to have a heart attack? Not at all. Whitehall I found there was an inverse relationship between status and cardiovascular disease. The lower a man's position and socioeconomic status, the more risk factors (smoking, obesity, sedentary lifestyle). The all-cause mortality in the lowest status was *three times* the mortality of the highest. Even after controlling for all risk factors, the mortality from heart disease was still twice as high in the lowest grades compared with the highest grades.

The difference? Perceived control over their work. The higher your grade, the more you can control the type and rate of work—and dump any overflow on the desk of the person below you.

Low perceived control, having an external locus of control, kills you.

The Whitehall II study began in 1985, and addressed the narrow focus of Whitehall I. It followed 10,308 women and men employed at the time by the British civil service. This is a longitudinal study. It has had many phases and is still continuing. It included women, broadened the range of conditions, and has demonstrated the same social gradient of disease and mortality in heart disease, some cancers, chronic lung disease, gastrointestinal disease, depression, suicide, sickness absence, back pain, and general feelings of ill health.

It has been known for decades that poverty kills you, that people in the lowest socioeconomic categories suffer more disease and reduced mortality. But here was an extension to that understanding: it's a gradient, it's not all or nothing, and it's as much about health as disease. Here is Antonovsky's continuum of health—the higher up the social gradient, the better your health (and therefore the lower your risk of disease), but the key parameter is control, or rather perceived control, a belief in your own ability to control your destiny.

Also speaking in the closing session of Congress 2017 was the New Zealand anaesthetist, Robin Youngson. He also believes that doctors must do more to change the world, and he advocates that the way to do this is by bringing compassion back into medicine and healthcare. In fact, he proposes that we bring the principles of positive psychology and flourishing into our own lives (as doctors) and that we practise with compassion for our patients. What does this do? It improves job satisfaction for doctors and improves outcomes for patients. Youngson cited a study of patients with advanced lung cancer, who were allocated either to aggressive medical management or palliative care. Palliative care involves management by doctors and health professionals who are trained in holistic, compassionate care, focused on helping people make sense of the last phase in their life, and take control of their remaining days or weeks. What the researchers found was perhaps surprising. The patients who were allocated to palliative care had lower levels of depression, were happier, and their treatment costs were (inevitably) much lower; yet they lived considerably longer than the aggressive treatment group.

In the past 3 years, more research has been published on population studies. In the MIDUS (Midlife in the United States) survey, researchers followed nearly 5000 midlife Americans and compared their experience of life trauma (either ACEs or traumatic experiences in adult life) with risk of mortality. They found that the greater the number of traumatic events, the greater the all-cause mortality. However, this effect disappeared in the presence of what the researchers called 'mastery'—a high sense of perceived control, 'beliefs in one's ability to influence circumstances and attain goals'. They found a dose-response relationship between number of traumatic life events and mortality risk, with the risk being highest in those with the most such events and the lowest levels of mastery, of self-belief. They proposed that intervention in the form of more adaptive and positive coping strategies (such as problem-solving and support-seeking) could increase the sense of mastery, develop the perception of control and an internal locus of control, and therefore reduce the mortality risk. They proposed that this could be achieved by offering psychological support in the form of cognitive behavioural therapy given in a primary care setting.

Martin Seligman, in his years of research into positive psychology, provides some evidence that this approach could be effective. His early research was into the 'learned hopelessness' that comes from exposure to ACEs. He progressed to 'learned optimism', the concept that strategies can be taught to reframe how we view the adverse event, the belief we hold about it, and the consequences that it brings (known as the 'ABC model'). In this way, we learn to develop a more optimistic viewpoint that we can take control of our circumstances.

'Disruption for Healthy Futures'

After Congress 2017, I took over from Michael Gabbett as Congress Lead Fellow, chairing the committee to plan the conference programme and invite proposed speakers. At a meeting of senior members of the College, it had been determined that the shared interest model for Congress was working, and that the task of the Congress Programme Committee was to disrupt the model of the conference further, to be even more challenging and appealing to our College members.

What better theme for the conference, then, than 'Disruption for Healthy Futures'? 'Disruptive innovation' is a term coined by Professor Clayton Christensen of Harvard Business School to describe the introduction of a wholly new concept into a business market—often one that is cheaper and more effective than the accepted norm, and therefore disrupts the market.

It has been proposed that the delivery of healthcare is ripe for disruption, as the delivery of medical services in recent decades has become more specialized and expensive, and less sustainable, while not meeting the health needs of the population.

There is no better international example of this than healthcare in the US.

There have been so many iterations of healthcare change over the last three decades (in many Western countries), each lauded as better than the last. What happened? Each iteration cost more than the last. If there were improvements, they were incremental—we made things a bit better. To change things radically in healthcare delivery is difficult, there are many barriers to revolutionary change ('revolutionary' in the positive sense of a dramatic change). Even evolutionary change can be difficult.

Remember the UK's RCGP's future vision for general practice in the UK by 2030 mentioned in Chapter 3? I see in it the seeds of disruption (and certainly some prospect of creating an environment that welcomes disruption). At the same time, I also note the aspiration to do things just a bit better. The length of a GP consultation in the UK is currently just under 10 minutes, on average. By 2030, the aim is at least 15 minutes.

After leaving the UK, I worked in general practice in New Zealand for a year, where the consultation times I worked to were 15 minutes. The extra 5 minutes takes some of the pressure off the consultation, but it doesn't allow us to shift to prevention. Nowadays in my specialist practice, I will often take 1½ hours for an initial assessment of clients, to cover all domains of their life and health.

The patients in the UK who participated in the RCGP's large survey were very clear what they wanted—they want to be treated as 'equal partners' and they 'don't want to be treated as a set of symptoms; they want to be treated as individuals'. More than this, 'Patients say they want to know how to look after themselves, to reduce the risk of developing serious health conditions, to spot the signs of illness, and to treat their symptoms before seeing a doctor.'

Achieving this will, of necessity, involve disruption. Medicine and healthcare are not technology, but technological advances will inevitably also disrupt how medicine is practised and healthcare delivered. If we were to horizon gaze as to where technology is likely to head by 2030, I suspect we would all get very excited and see all sorts of incredible advances. Technology is advancing exponentially. If we were to apply the same thinking to medicine and general practice, I suspect we would come up with many different and exciting scenarios. I absolutely respect the process that the RCGP has followed, and the motivation behind it, but I strongly suspect that, by 2030, general practice, primary care, and indeed the practice of medicine will look very different to the future vision painted by the RCGP.

One of the factors likely to impact the future of medicine is climate change. Climate change is both a stimulus of the need for disruption in how we deliver healthcare and also a disruptor itself, but in the negative sense. Congress in 2018 was opened by an oration by Dr David Pencheon, lead for the NHS Sustainable Development Unit (England). His topic was 'Disruption: a route to better health and care' and he pointed out that for healthcare to be sustainable, disruption has to occur. The delivery of care has to be sustainable in terms of the world's finite resources and our need to take into account the environmental impact of our actions. Dr Pencheon drew our attention to a leading editorial in *The BMJ* which warned that climate change is a health emergency. Not only must we act now to mitigate the effects of climate change, but we have to act now in terms of preparing healthcare systems for the adverse impacts on health which will inevitably occur.

Who needs to do something about it? Clearly governments do, and healthcare policymakers. Challenging the audience, Dr Pencheon pointed out that doctors are important influencers in society, and we each have individual responsibility. 'We're all leaders. Get used to it!'

After 2½ days of engaging with and challenging over 1000 specialist doctors and specialists in training, the final session of Congress was again billed as the highlight. It was a daunting prospect for the team running Congress—it was ambitious and very different from a traditional conference session. The 2-hour session opened with the stage in darkness, and a spotlight came on ... revealing a solitary patient, telling the story of her life. Mary wasn't really a patient, she was an actor, but as the scene unfolded, Mary told the story of her life and her health from birth, through childhood, through bad decisions in adolescence, to adversity, illness, and finally gastric cancer. At every stage of the way, the story was punctuated by presentations by specialist paediatricians and physicians of the RACP. Each touched Mary's life for a brief period and helped her deal with that brush with illness and disease, but her life went on. Each time, there was more to happen. In fact, just for an added touch of authenticity, we even included a police superintendent in full uniform. Superintendent Luke Freudenstein works with young people in a district of Sydney. He played his role very convincingly as he described how he had worked with Mary during her troubled teen years to get her involved in sport, encouraging her to make better life choices.

The session was to introduce the concept of life course theory, the topic of the following year's Congress. Life course theory identifies the different facets that make up our lives from birth, and how our social context and the choices we make at every step of the way affect what happens next in our lives: our education, relationships, life decisions, health, and disease experiences. And for the specialist doctors in the audience, it was to remind them of the influences of everything that has happened to their patient up to that point, and that we only touch our patients' lives for a brief time.

The final speaker was Dr George Laking, Chair of the RACP's Māori Health Committee. George Laking is an oncologist, and he presented his role in looking after Mary's gastric cancer. He spoke of palliative care and the role of spirituality in palliative care and end-of-life care. He told us of the importance of spirituality to Māori people, and the role of nature and the land (very important to the indigenous people of Australia too, the Aboriginal and Torres Strait Islander people). He described how spirituality is incorporated into the Māori model of health, 'te whare tapa whā'. But he also alluded to the fact that we all have a belief system of some kind. Consideration of a broader definition of spirituality, as used in palliative care, needs to be considered for the health of us all.

We are one

The theme of the RACP Congress in 2019 was 'Impacting Health Along the Life Course'. It recognized that as doctors in the RACP we cover many different specialties, from paediatrics and child health to every system in the body, to public health, including my own speciality, occupational and environmental medicine, and that each of us touches the lives of our patients.

Early 2019 had been a difficult time for New Zealanders, especially the people of Christchurch, with the devastating events of the mosque shootings of 15 March in which 51 people lost their lives. Planned to incite hatred, the events of that day achieved the opposite: the tragedy brought communities together. The national remembrance service held in Christchurch exactly a fortnight later had the title 'Ko Tātou, Tātou', a Māori phrase meaning 'We are one'.

As I gave my welcome speech at the start of Congress, I explained that as the Congress programme had come together, this expression had become significant for me; the realization that as doctors and patients, we are one. We are all connected by the same hopes and fears, and we all have a journey of life that we progress through. If patients' lives and health are affected by the events and choices of their lives, then exactly the same applies for doctors. We tend to forget this. We are one.

I had signed up to lead two Congress events. For me, Sydney was the dress rehearsal for what I had envisaged for Congress in Auckland in May 2019. Further disruption of the conference model was planned. One instance was the incorporation of Māori tikanga (Māori protocol, the way of doing things right) throughout Congress, including frequent use of the Māori language, and the opening with a pōwhiri (Māori welcoming ceremony) and opening and closing of Congress with a Māori prayer, or karakia. We were therefore thrilled and honoured to have the opening oration delivered by Sir Mason Durie. Sir Mason is a Māori doctor who specialized in psychiatry, but is best known for his work as professor of Māori studies and his contribution to the health of Māori, and indeed to our understanding of health in its broadest sense.

In his 1985 paper, 'A Māori perspective of health', Sir Mason contrasted the way that Māori culture views health with the Western viewpoint. He noted that the WHO definition of health included the physical, psychological, and social domains of life, but for Māori this definition missed one important domain. In fact, it is the most important domain of all to Māori—spiritual health. He presented these four domains as being the cornerstones of life, traditionally shown as the four cornerstones of a house, translated from the Māori, te whare tapa whā, now known as the Māori model of health.

Sir Mason's oration is inspirational to watch.[4] Sir Mason tells the story of how, as a young and eager junior hospital doctor in 1964, he first encountered a way of seeing health and illness that was very different from what he was being taught. He described the story of a very ill young girl whose only carer was her koro, her grandfather. Sir Mason contrasted the traditional wisdom of the Māori elder with his own training in science, Western medicine, and realized that there were different perspectives which are all valid and relevant. But we omit that cultural dimension from healthcare delivery at our peril. He gave us five lessons from that 1964 encounter to consider:

1. It is time now for medicine to discount the seventeenth-century model of Cartesian duality that says that the body and the mind are separate. The two are inextricably linked.
2. We need to understand and acknowledge the connection between our health and our environment, both negative and positive—the connection between ourselves and nature.
3. The importance of whānau, the family, for our health and intergenerational transfer of knowledge and experience. (In Māori, the word for family is whānau, which denotes an extended view of the immediate family and those who connect to the family, since community elders have an important influence in the life of the family.)
4. A need to recognize spirituality as an important part of our journey to wellbeing.
5. The need to work with two bodies of knowledge: scientific and cultural.

Science has its place, but we mustn't be blinded to the fact that there are different knowledge systems which view life and health from very different perspectives. Medical science views health and illness through the microscope, looking at finer and finer detail, but may be missing the big picture. Cultural (indigenous) belief systems do the opposite—they go outwards from the illness to look at the full context of the individual, their family, and their environment. A holistic viewpoint: we are more than the sum of our parts.

Sir Mason left us with the thought that doctors sit at the interface of medical science and cultural knowledge. This creates challenges, but more importantly, opportunities. The opportunities are for a more holistic practice of medicine that incorporates mind, body, and spirit, that views a person in the context of their whole lives, including their family and their environment. An understanding of health that considers how the socioeconomic circumstances relate to the diagnosis, and values the combination of clinical and cultural factors and the role of family, elders, and intergenerational links.

As he left the stage, he said to me, 'I hope it's still relevant.' I replied, 'Not only is it still relevant for Māori, but it's relevant for all New Zealanders.'

What I didn't realize, until I reread his original 1985 paper, was that he already knew that.

Of course, this isn't just about Māori, it is about all of us. Back in 1985, Sir Mason had said:

The limitations of contemporary health services, particularly in the spiritual dimension, are increasingly acknowledged by many senior health administrators throughout the country and the incorporation of Māori attitudes and Māori experts into Western health systems should lead to a more comprehensive approach to health problems in New Zealand.[5]

The logic and eloquence with which he presented these views to a Congress with nearly 1000 specialist, traditional Western doctors was resounding. The satisfaction rating score given by the audience for the presentation was 4.6 out of 5, the highest of the many presentations at Congress. We were persuaded by the logic.

This set the scene for a Congress that was greeted with high levels of satisfaction. There was one more disruption of the traditional conference delivery model awaiting the audience: 'Doctors Got Talent'. Before the audience were allowed to rush off to morning tea, one of our own specialist doctors took to the stage, and sang his rendition of Frank Sinatra's song 'My Way'. He did a great job, and was applauded enthusiastically. Throughout Congress we showcased the talents of doctors—in their music, poetry, writing, art, and photography. To show that doctors have lives and interests outside work, to demonstrate that doctors are people too.

The shared interest sessions brought together the concepts that would impact any of the doctors present. In 'The life course paradigm—the key to unlocking optimal health' we considered the interrelationship between our patients' health and their life course; the circumstances and events that have led them to the illness that presents to the paediatricians and physicians of the RACP, and the likelihood that that they would return to the childhood poverty and poor housing and joblessness which held the roots of their illness in the first place.

In 'Obesity: rising to the challenge' we considered the impact of diet and lifestyle on the epidemic of obesity, diabetes, cardiovascular disease, and mental ill health. For me, the star of the show was former professional boxer Dave 'Brown Buttabean' Letele. He told the story of his realization that he was unhappy being an obese boxer and how he took it into his own hands to do something about it and lose 90 kg. Now he runs bootcamps for the people of Auckland, many of them overweight Māori and Pacific people. His 'Buttabean Motivation' bootcamps encourage people to take the first small steps to improving their nutrition and activity. By starting with small steps, he achieves amazing results, with many people achieving a weight loss of 50 kg or more. Over 25,000 kg has been lost by people attending his camps.

In 'The first 1000 days—the window of opportunity for long term health', our speakers considered the evidence that the roots of health and disease are very significantly influenced by the circumstances of the first thousand days of life. New Zealand leads the world in terms of research into the effect of life circumstances on health, disease, wellbeing, and social outcomes, through a number of studies, including the world-renowned Dunedin Study. This study follows the 1000 babies born in the New Zealand city of Dunedin over 12 months in 1972–1973. Most of these individuals continue to have their health and social circumstances tracked to the present day. The information we have gained from the study about how the circumstances of where we're born, grown, school, live, and work (the social determinants of health) impact disease processes and how our lives turn out is staggering. This body of research has contributed significantly to the science of epigenetics, how environment modifies the expression of our genes.

We continued our exploration of the impact of medically unexplained symptoms. I facilitated a masterclass with specialist medical input as well as physiotherapy and psychology input. Key messages were that it is important to do two things for patients with these conditions; first, listen empathically, and second, let them know that their symptoms are very real. There are positive messages about how they can be managed, with the evidence base identifying two particular modalities: graded exercise and cognitive behavioural therapy.

Other sessions dealt with the need for partnership and integrated care, and the opioid epidemic (and the role of doctors), but the highlight was billed to be the final session, which was a 2-hour exploration of the health of doctors, titled 'Physician, heal thyself'. This was presented by doctors at various stages of their careers, from junior doctor to the pre-retirement stage of the RACP President, Professor Mark Lane. I must confess to some nepotism in planning this session, since the junior doctor was my son, Matt Beaumont. Matt opened by recounting his experience of transitioning from medical student to junior doctor, and how he dealt with the pressure and looked after his own health and wellbeing. Each of the doctors spoke of the challenges of having a medical career and juggling the events of life.

We explored the concept of the need for doctors to look after themselves better, to prioritize their own health, and to recognize that doctors have a life course too. If we need to apply compassion to the care of our patients, then we also need to apply compassion to our own health. Dr Sam Hazledine made the point that it is essential for doctors to look after their own health, because if they don't, they are not in a good position to look after their patients. Ill doctors provide poor care.

There's an insidious illness that many doctors suffer from, that of burnout. Burnout occurs particularly in doctors because of the kind of people we are. We care about people, we are very devoted to what we do, and because of that we tend to disregard our own health and needs. A 2016 survey of senior New Zealand doctors found that nearly 50 per cent were suffering one or more of the three symptoms of burnout: emotional exhaustion, cynicism or compassion fatigue, and doubt that one is making a difference.[6] This finding is seen around the world.

Dr Sam Hazledine has devoted his career to improving the lives of doctors. He took the case to the World Medical Association that the Declaration of Geneva (the modern Hippocratic oath) should include doctors' health and wellbeing. The revision he proposed was incorporated in 2017, and the relevant section reads, 'I will attend to my own health, well-being, and abilities in order to provide care of the highest standard'.[7] Prior to that time, the focus was purely on the responsibility of doctors towards their patients and colleagues. Here was the recognition that we need to care for ourselves first. Put on our own oxygen mask before helping others with theirs.

As I gave the closing comments and farewell for Congress, I reminded the audience that the theme was about the role that doctors play in impacting the life and health of their patients. Having closed with the session on the life course of doctors, I reminded them of the subtheme I had introduced: 'ko tātou, tātou' (we are one). Our patients deserve to be treated as people, but doctors are people too.

As I delivered my final sentence, the emotion and power of the event struck me, and I had tears in my eyes as I said, 'Remember, every healthcare interaction involves a person with their own life story treating a person with their own life story.'

7

How to Reclaim Your Life

It's time to pull all the themes together. It's been a few years now since the model came to me. My life journey had taken me through the recognition that something wasn't working with the model of medical practice I had been taught, having seen thousands of patients who had been failed by the system. I then had my own experience of being on the receiving end as a patient and realizing that to claim back my life demanded a lot more than the things my doctors had done for me, as well meaning and caring as they had been.

I was on the early morning flight from Sydney. Thoughts were drifting round my mind as to how to take this experience, this realization, into practice. Then it hit me.

'Yes!' I exclaimed out loud. The businessman next to me jumped awake.

'What's happened?'

I explained the pieces of the jigsaw had just fallen into place for me, I had just seen the basis for a new model of medical practice.

He said, 'Tell me about it.' So I did.

It didn't take long, and he got it instantly. He said, 'I want some of that. In fact, my brother needs you. He's a lawyer. Just been through a marital separation. Lost his way. Doesn't know where he's going in life. He's illness waiting to happen.'

When I got home, I told my son, Matt, then a medical student. (I have described him as the wisest man I know.) He said, 'Dad, if it helps just one person, and that person is you, then it's been worthwhile.'

My daughter, Emma, was home from university, with three of her mates. They wanted to hear about it too. They said, 'Wow, that would work for us too! We want to stay fit and healthy!'

An empowerment model for patients works at whatever level you need it to work, whatever age you are. It also fits with being a prevention model. But first I need to explain prevention further.

Positive Medicine. David Beaumont, Oxford University Press. © Oxford University Press 2021.
DOI: 10.1093/oso/9780192845184.003.0008

Employment, poverty, and health

In medicine, we talk about prevention being on three levels: primary, secondary, and tertiary. Primary prevention is just as you might expect: preventing ill health and promoting health. Secondary prevention is spotting problems early, as they are occurring, and intervening early to prevent them developing or to reverse the process. Tertiary prevention occurs when illness and disease have already developed, and the doctor acts to mitigate the effects, allowing the person to get on with their life, despite any disability caused by the condition. Although the goal is to shift prevention to an earlier and earlier stage, which usually means younger in life, the good news is that prevention and enhancement of health and wellbeing can occur at any age and in any circumstances, any level of illness or disability.

This also fits with the new definition of health, that health is the ability to adapt and self-manage in the face of life's challenges. We all face life's challenges (with some individuals getting more than their fair share), but with support, coaching, and planning we can all learn techniques to take control of our lives and adapt to be able to get the most out of our lives. We can learn how to develop an internal locus of control—the belief that we can control our own destinies and live life with meaning and purpose. The research shows that by developing an internal locus of control, we statistically increase our chances of living longer with less illness and disease.

The social gradient of health says that the better your social circumstances, the more control you take over the social determinants of health, and the more your health and life expectancy will improve. And that is true at any point of the gradient, so we can all improve our life outcomes by taking control. But what has this got to do with doctors? According to Sir Harry Burns, Sir Michael Marmot, and Dr David Pencheon, everything! Doctors are looked to by patients for guidance as to what they need to do to overcome disease and stay healthy; it's the role that doctors play in society. ('We're all leaders, get used to it!')

After Sir Harry Burns' presentation at Congress, and the exhortation of Sir Michael Marmot that doctors must do more to change the world, a group of us got together. We put it to the Policy and Advocacy Committee of our College that the RACP needed to provide leadership to the rest of the medical profession as to what role doctors should play in helping their patients take control of the social determinants of health, and how we can truly influence change in the world. We reviewed the world literature on the subject and found that there is a lot of opinion that says doctors must accept they have a role to play, and contribute to positive change in the world. The four occupational physicians in the team were surprised to see that the role of employment, one of the main opportunities for helping people take control of their social circumstances, had not been particularly emphasized in other literature. Paid work is one of the key factors in helping people escape the poverty trap. Not to take away from the value of unpaid voluntary work, or the role of non-working parents, the evidence is clear—good work is good for health, and employment underpins the strategy for people to address so many of the social determinants of health.

On behalf of the RACP, we produced a guidance document called *Employment, Poverty and Health*, which I launched publicly at Congress 2019.[1] It identifies seven areas where doctors can influence the social determinants of health:

Employment—promoting the health benefits of good work to patients and employers.

Models of healthcare delivery—contributing to innovative and patient-centred models of healthcare.

Leadership—doctors leading by example through their own clinical practice.

Advocacy—advocating for policies which address the social determinants of health.

Collaboration—collaborating with others to address social determinants and promote good work.

Teaching and learning—imparting clinical knowledge to students, trainees, and colleagues.

Research—contributing to the evidence base of the health effects of the social determinants of health.

As an example of how doctors can influence through advocacy, I was proud to be involved in a piece of advocacy work undertaken by the New Zealand Committee of the RACP. Just prior to the country's general election, we produced an 'election statement' that we sent to all political parties. Under the campaign hashtag #MakeItTheNorm, we urged politicians and political parties to make health equity the norm in New Zealand. We cited examples of where health inequity is linked to the social determinants of health, and the terrible effects this has on the health of our patients (and therefore all New Zealanders), with Māori and Pacific people being heavily over-represented in the adverse statistics. We focused on three areas:

- Making healthy housing the norm.
- Making good work the norm.
- Making whānau (family) wellbeing the norm.

We gave examples of simple policy changes that would enable this shift in equity. Our statement gained considerable traction with the media. Importantly, our own College members recognized the importance of doctors taking a moral and ethical stance and stepping up to provide leadership. We received many messages of support from colleagues.

The circumstances in which we are born, raised, and educated are to a large extent out of our control, since in our early (and most formative) years we are dependent on our parents. There are many inspiring stories of people from backgrounds of poverty who have taken control of their own destiny and gone on to have lives of great meaning and purpose. One of the limiting factors is the learned hopelessness that dooms people to live lives of hardship, poverty, and challenge which leads to ill health and reduced mortality. There is much that doctors, the healthcare system, and also the education system can do to encourage and teach principles and coping strategies to learn the optimism that there are many aspects of our destiny we can take control of. As the serenity prayer says, it takes serenity to accept the things one cannot change, courage to change the things one can, and wisdom to know the difference. That's the potential touch point for doctors: helping people gain the wisdom to know the difference and develop the courage to act.

But superimposed on top of these circumstances are the curve balls that life throws at all of us, the adversity that comes in the form of accidents, illness, family tragedies, relationship breakdown, and the death of loved ones. Sadly, we all encounter such events at some points in our lives, and some people seem to get more than their fair share. Because my assessment of clients involves a comprehensive review of all aspects of their lives, I ask them about personal traumatic experiences. I feel privileged and humbled at the extent that people are prepared to discuss with me the most private and sensitive parts of their life. It astounds me the extent to which life brings adversity and the degree to which people are resilient and get on with their lives. One such person had a long string of adverse events, one of which was the death of his wife and son in a car accident. Later in the assessment he referred to the death of his wife and daughter, which confused me.

He said, 'Oh, sorry, yes, that was my first wife and daughter. My second wife and son were also killed in a car accident.'

What a dreadful set of circumstances. Yet he was really quite matter of fact about the events, and had remarried and had another child. The words 'What doesn't kill us makes us stronger' (attributed to the German philosopher Nietzsche) have been demonstrated to be true time and time again. Some people have the ability to pick themselves up after adversity, dust themselves down, and get on with life and become more resilient for it. It's termed 'post-traumatic growth'.

What sets these people apart is their internal locus of control—the belief they have in their own ability to take control of their lives. One specific life challenge that doctors see all the time is, of course, illness, particularly serious illness. Probably the most extreme example of internal locus of control I have encountered was a woman who was referred to me for a return-to-work programme after she had been off work for 12 months, having had acute pancreatitis. She had experienced the most severe form of the condition, had been in and out of intensive care, had had several operations to drain abscesses, had been fed with a feeding tube for months on end, and had lost nearly half her body weight. I knew the assessment was going to be a challenge, but I wasn't prepared for why.

I started the assessment by introducing myself and explaining my role, but before I could finish, she interrupted me. 'You can stop right there. I'm telling you now that there's nothing you can say or do that will stop me going back to work.'

Her expectation was that I would say that she wasn't fit for work, but she was the most determined client I've ever met. We were able to put in place measures to support her and work with her employer to achieve a successful return to work. Her determination meant that failure was never likely. She was in complete control, despite all the setbacks she had endured.

I met another person with an internal locus of control, but who instead had misunderstood the power he held for his own destiny. He hadn't worked for 20 years after a relatively minor back injury. He was my age but looked much older. He walked like an old man and used a walking stick. He, too, interrupted my introduction, and said, 'You're wasting your time and mine. I've told them I'm not going back to work. I took them to court and won. I told them I would never go back to work and I haven't!'

I asked him one question. 'What is your quality of life like?'

'Oh, dreadful,' he replied, 'I can't do anything, so I just watch television all day.' He didn't get the irony that, although he had chosen to take control of his own life, he had resisted all attempts to support him back to work and in doing so had chosen a life of limited function and disability. His life could have been very, very different.

He was right, there was no point trying to change his mind. He had a fixed mindset and he had set his destiny in stone.

The role of childhood trauma

Many of the clients I see have an external locus of control. They believe that their fate lies outside themselves, that their destiny is influenced by circumstances or by other people. When I ask them what they want to happen next, they often say, 'I just want someone to fix me.'

Many of them have learned hopelessness. Their lack of belief and faith in their own ability to take control has developed as a result of circumstances, and often those circumstances are also at the root of their illness. What those circumstances are will vary from person to person, but they usually surface at some point in our connections. Often, it's to do with childhood influences, but it can be at any point in life and any set of circumstances. The common theme is that the experiences are traumatic (either brief and short term, or persistent and enduring) and usually the person (especially if they were still a child) was powerless to do anything about it.

It astounds me how many people I see for chronic pain problems who have experienced childhood sexual abuse. Often this has either not been identified, or the link between the abuse and the subsequent development of chronic pain has not been made. As we have discussed in Chapter 6, ACEs are a significant risk factor for later adult illness and disease, including chronic pain. And they are sadly very common. The Dunedin Study found that 30 per cent of the female participants and 9 per cent of the males had experienced some form of child sexual abuse.[2]

Data from the 2016 National Survey of Children's Health (NSCH) identified that 45 per cent of children in the US had experienced at least one ACE, with 10 per cent experiencing three or more, a marker for very high risk of disease and early mortality.[3] The fear and hopelessness these circumstances create can put the body into a state of chronic arousal of the neuroendocrine system, as I described in Chapter 5, and upset the body's normal corrective mechanism, homeostasis. The resulting allostatic load increases the levels of cortisol and decreases the sensitivity of the tissues' response to that cortisol, increasing inflammatory markers and putting the body in a chronic state of arousal and inflammation. On the scale of ease to dis-ease, many of these people are in a state of dis-ease, a state of fear and constant vigilance for threat. This is why the brain is in defensive mode and overinterprets normal signals as being noxious and painful.

Chronic pain can occur after injury, particularly in a person in a state of disease, but it can also occur as part of medically unexplained symptoms such as fibromyalgia. In his book, *The Fibro Fix*, Dr David Brady gives a really helpful description of the underlying mechanism in fibromyalgia which, he explains, is a centrally mediated disorder (central sensitization disorder):

> *Centrally mediated* means that the pain originates from a dysfunction in the central nervous system, which is made up of the brain and spinal cord. In other words, fibromyalgia is a disorder involving the way the nervous system *processes* pain. … A glitch in your central nervous system causes your body to process pain in an over-sensitized way and misinterpret the signals it receives.[4]

Brady highlights the research that demonstrates that children exposed to ACEs are 2.7 times more likely to develop conditions such as fibromyalgia and chronic fatigue syndrome. Because fibromyalgia is 'medically unexplained', it can be difficult to tackle such issues with sufferers.

In a response to Dr Brady's online blog, SR responded, 'Thank you for writing this in this way. When I heard fibromyalgia linked to childhood trauma in the past, it always sounded like another version of "it's all in your head" because the physical basis was not explained. It was said as if the fibromyalgia is a psychological symptom rather than a physiological process. This explanation makes it easier for me to accept this link.' KS wrote, 'This article gives me hope in my positive advancement towards managing healing and repairing my mind and body.'[5]

Like me, Dr Brady is unclear as to the value of counselling in such cases. He points out that unless it is delivered as part of a specific therapy, there may be a risk that bringing up very painful issues results in a tendency to dwell on them. Where serious childhood trauma is identified, I would certainly recommend assessment by a clinical psychologist. But I would caution against long-term counselling if it is not focused on helping the person move forward with their life and heal from the experience, rather than keep reliving it. (I have sometimes encountered counsellors holding back clients from moving on with their lives, arguing *against* helping people get back to work.)

Empowerment

Cameron was referred to me by his insurance company for a positive medicine programme. He had been off work for 6 months with diagnoses of fibromyalgia and chronic fatigue syndrome. At the time, he was 23. He had widespread pain and muscular tenderness, and was sleeping about 20 hours a day. I obtained copies of his investigation results from his GP. He had been thoroughly investigated and all test results were normal. There was a history of overseas travel shortly prior to development of symptoms, so he had been referred to an infectious diseases specialist consultant to test for tropical infection. Further investigations excluded this possibility, and the consultant reached a diagnosis of fibromyalgia and chronic fatigue syndrome, with a history of a viral infection probably the trigger.

When I saw Cameron for assessment, I agreed he met the criteria for the diagnoses; yet even careful probing did not identify a clear history of viral illness. Certainly, post-viral fatigue is common after specific viruses such as glandular fever (infectious mononucleosis) and influenza. But there is no evidence to implicate a specific viral cause for fibromyalgia, though doctors seem to be very keen to try to identify such a cause for many of the clients I see. Cameron's case was interesting, because the only 'trauma' I could identify was self-imposed. He is a very driven and determined young man. As well as working full-time as an orchard worker, he was also renovating his house. Having bought his own house, he was coming home from a full day of heavy work and working long into the evening to get the house ready for himself and his girlfriend. His body ached, and he was constantly tired, but he continued to push through. It is not surprising that he had put his body and mind into a defensive mode, a state of dis-ease and chronically activated nervous system. It is easy to see how the frequent aching and pushing through set up a pain cycle which led to overstimulation of the brain's defence systems and a central sensitization disorder.

I worked through the four domains of the cornerstones of his health with him—physical, psychological, emotional, and spiritual. There were a number of good prognostic markers (i.e. indictors for a good outcome), including those that had led to the condition in the first instance. As a highly motivated and determined person, Cameron has a strong sense of self-belief and therefore an internal locus of control. The referral had come from the insurance company at an early stage (sadly, I am often only referred clients after they have been off work for a matter of many months or years). Early intervention is the best way to achieve a good outcome. And the trauma which had sensitized the mind–body connection was very recent (and not from childhood, for instance). Cameron was a delight to work with; he was very clear what he wanted to achieve. He wanted to get off the medication, get back to work, and get on with his life. He was very receptive to the modalities I advised. The key was to allow his body to get back into balance, to allow an opportunity for his body to heal and to revert to homeostasis: to go from its state of dis-ease to ease.

We put in place a multidisciplinary programme, with me, a physiotherapist, an occupational therapist, and a psychologist. My role was overseeing the process and working with Cameron to reduce his pain medication. (To be clear, the commonest role I take in advising on pain medication is to reduce and rationalize it as quickly as I can.) Together with the occupational therapist, I also liaised with his employer at the orchard. His boss was very supportive, both of Cameron and of the process (as I'm sure you can imagine, he was well regarded as a good worker). He allowed us to use the orchard to simulate work activities very carefully and gradually, rather than needing to get Cameron into the gym for a physio-supervised gym programme.

The occupational therapist worked with Cameron to structure his day and gradually increase his function, to ensure that he fitted in his programme with the rest of his life activities, encouraging him to reconnect with family and friends. We also involved his girlfriend, to ensure that she understood the process and could appropriately support Cameron. The psychologist only needed a couple of sessions with him, to help him understand the mechanisms that were occurring in his brain and body and how he could take control of them. Cameron was a quick learner and she was impressed with his character. The occupational therapist also worked with him on sleep hygiene, the process of gradually returning his sleep pattern to normal. Excessive sleep and rest in chronic fatigue syndrome is counterproductive. ('Too much sleep makes you tired.') It can also perpetuate a cycle of losing fitness and becoming deconditioned, which makes sufferers feel less and less able to participate in activity: a vicious cycle.

Over the next 2 months, Cameron gradually increased the work activities at the orchard, to the extent that he was doing useful work, but on reduced hours. He was off all pain relief, and his sleep was coming back to normal. That's when he announced that he had other plans for work. His real goal, what he really wanted to do, was landscape gardening! Clearly that is a very heavy job and an ambitious goal for someone in the recovery stage from illness. A month later, I phoned Cameron for a catch-up discussion. I could hear the smile on his face over the phone. (Have you noticed how you can tell when someone is smiling even over the phone?) It was a beautiful summer's day in Central Otago, and he said, 'I'm in a garden in Wanaka, doing my dream job.'

Three years later, just a few weeks ago, I bumped into him and his girlfriend in the supermarket. Grinning, they told me they had recently got married.

Cameron is still working in landscape gardening and doing really well. He confirmed he was happy for me to recount his case, and to use his real name.

Cameron's case illustrates really well how an empowerment model of health works. He was the ideal candidate for it. He readily accepted that the outcome was under his control, his responsibility, and that the benefits of success were available to him. As the team working with him, we consciously gave him the power, we involved him (and often his girlfriend) in every decision, and we respected his viewpoint. But all we did was *facilitate* his healing, his shift from dis-ease to ease. From illness to health; the ability to adapt and self-manage in the face of life's challenges. The more I've worked with people like Cameron, the more I've realized that often, the answer is within. They know intuitively what they should be doing, and my job becomes simply to facilitate them to listen to their own intuition, and to help them pull the plan together.

How the body heals itself

The concept of the body healing itself is one that is often portrayed in the wellbeing literature. I asked my son Matt what he thought about me mentioning it in this book, from the perspective of a doctor reading it.

I was a little surprised by his response, because he said, 'Phew . . . I wouldn't do it; it sounds a bit alternative.'

That means I've got to tackle it head-on!

Here's the statement: the body heals itself, and every doctor is taught this. In fact, to believe any different flies in the face of everything we are taught as doctors. The human body is a truly remarkable healing machine, and all that doctors and medical science do is to facilitate that. We go wrong when we forget that and try to do too much, do more harm than good, and sometimes kill patients in the process.

What happens when we cut ourselves? If we cut ourselves cleanly with a knife, the body mounts its immediate healing mechanism and we heal by what is called 'primary intention'. If the laceration is more complicated, or tissue has been excised or is brought together after a delay, the body heals by 'secondary intention'. A bigger healing response is mounted, with a greater inflammatory component, more immune cells brought into play, and more fibrous tissue involved. But we heal. Break a bone, fix it in position, it heals. If it's not straight, the body does what it can to straighten it—the process of remodelling. Remarkable!

Infection? Sure, for the last few decades we've had antibiotics. What do antibiotics do? They help give the body a fighting advantage against bacteria, but it's still the body's defence system that does the healing. In immune deficiency syndromes, there comes a point when the body's defence system has been so depleted that no amount of antibiotics is going to make a difference. The fight is lost. It's only in the course of the last century that we've had specific drugs to tackle specific deficiencies in the body's own defences, such as the use of allopurinol to block the production of uric acid, to prevent the formation of uric acid crystals that cause gout.

Doctors have been a respected and integral part of our society, globally, for millennia. What did doctors do before antibiotics and allopurinol? They were *healers*. They facilitated their patients' ability to heal themselves. The first of the modern doctors was Hippocrates, 2500 years ago. He was the first person to investigate the course of illness, to determine the prognosis or likely outcome. But his main advice was to focus on adequate rest and nutrition and for the doctor to do more observing than treating (we call this 'watchful waiting'). As a doctor, he was the first of the modern healers!

What about the drugs the pre-modern doctors dispensed? To a very great extent, there was no evidence base for their efficacy. But they worked—at least to some extent. For many drugs that were prescribed, the doctors believed that they would work. They worked it out by trial and error—the empirical method—even though we can look back now and say that there is no evidence they should work. But there was another class of drugs, ones that the doctor knew shouldn't work, because there was no active ingredient. But they worked anyway; medicine's best-kept secret—the placebo effect.

When I was doing my GP training in England, I was allocated to a tiny village practice in rural Derbyshire. The elderly GP had taken over the practice from his father. In the consulting room were three large glass containers, one containing green liquid, another red, and the third orange. The GP explained they were a relic from his father's practice that he kept because they looked impressive and were a reminder of medical practice from a previous era. He explained they contained different coloured dyes and flavouring, but there was no active ingredient. But one was dispensed as a tonic, another for dry cough, and the third for loose cough. They were overtly placebos. Dispensed by the doctor when he believed that there was no other treatment he could give that was likely to be effective, they gave the body an opportunity to heal.

But there is evidence that placebos do more than that. In trials of many different conditions, placebo medication will often produce a 15–30 per cent improvement in symptoms.[6] This is a real nuisance for pharmaceutical companies, because in conducting the gold standard for clinical trials, randomized controlled trials, the active drug being tested is often compared to an inert alternative, and the trial participants are not told whether they are being given the trial drug or the inert one. Unfortunately (for the research team), often the patients given the inert drug show a significant improvement in symptoms because of the placebo effect. It is also likely that the therapeutic effect of many drugs in common use is due significantly to the placebo effect, particularly drugs used in pain relief and antidepressants. (In fact, there is good evidence that antidepressants are either no better than placebo or only marginally so.) Even so-called sham surgery in the form of (fake) arthroscopic surgery for osteoarthritis of the knee has been shown to be equally as effective as true surgery. The EVOLVE project of the RACP has identified many such therapies, throughout the many different specialties, which are either no better than placebo, or even cause harm.

'Placebo' comes from the Latin words meaning 'I will please'. We have identified that the opposite is also true; hence the term 'nocebo' or 'I will harm'. The nocebo effect occurs when a doctor tells a patient that a side effect is likely to occur, and it does; even if later it is found that the information was wrong, or the drug dose was so low that it wouldn't have been expected to cause any effect at all. It is also true when a doctor tells a patient that he's 'likely to end up in a wheelchair', or that she's 'never going to work again'. The power of those statements acts as a nocebo, and can create a self-fulfilling prophesy.

If doctors used to prescribe placebos before so-called evidence-based drugs were available, does it still happen? And if not, should it?

In researching for this section, I came across a provocative article called 'Why don't we exploit the hell out of the placebo effect?' Isn't that a great question? If an inert tablet, with no active ingredient and no side effects, can produce a significant benefit in symptoms, why don't doctors prescribe them regularly?

The answer is that many do. In 2016, in a large survey of GPs in the UK, 97 per cent admitted to using placebos: either drugs that they knew were not indicated for their active component, or inert tablets, such as sugar pills.[7] The majority of GPs believed it was ethical to do so in certain circumstances. The German Medical Association has gone further, and recommended to doctors that they should prescribe placebos if they believe it may help and if there is no safe alternative.

In an additional twist, there is some research that suggests that even 'honest placebos' have a beneficial effect; that is, when a patient is given a placebo and told, 'This is a placebo, it contains no active ingredient.' There is evidence also that as well as patient belief being important (in the case of the 'honest placebo' maybe even a subconscious and conditioned belief), an important factor is the way the placebo is prescribed by the doctor. An empathetic or compassionate doctor has been shown to be more likely to prescribe a placebo. This adds weight to the concept that Michael Balint described, of 'the drug, doctor'. As doctors, we need to recognize the powerful effect for good we can have, and acknowledge the positive effect we have on the healing of our patients. But we also need to recognize the flip side that power brings—the nocebo effect, which is iatrogenesis, inadvertent harm caused by doctors.

Don't get me wrong. It would be ungrateful of me not to acknowledge the wonders of modern medicine, and the amazing technological advances. I am very grateful for my two new hips. I am grateful for the care I received when I had my heart attack. If I had been told I needed a coronary artery stent or bypass graft I would have said, 'Bring it on!' I take my aspirin and my statin with enthusiasm every morning and evening. But the medical model is not enough, and we now have very, very good evidence of what we could be doing to truly influence the health of our patients. I know, from the satisfaction ratings from RACP Congress, from the thousand or so specialist physicians and paediatricians who attended, that doctors are ready to listen and want to know more.

The doctor as human being

Many people tell me they have the best GP in the world. They can't have, because I've got him already! The concept of a new model of practice will not be for everyone; apart from anything else, the healthcare system is not set up to allow doctors to practise more holistically. We need specialists, we need ultra-specialists, we need medical advances. It may be that the more technical the branch of medicine, the more the doctor needs to practise to the medical model—though more compassion in healthcare can only benefit patients and doctors.

I recently went with my partner to see her doctor. It was important I didn't let on I was a doctor too. She has recently developed a chronic illness and has suffered dreadfully from the symptoms. Sadly, she has been in a place of chronic stress, and the roots of the illness are clear.

The start of the consultation was a predictable review of medication and advice about optimizing timing and dosage. Then the GP stopped. She sighed and said:

What a dreadful time you have had. The symptoms are awful and so debilitating. What I want you to believe is that there is light at the end of the tunnel. The likelihood is that you will get on top of this, and there is every chance that you will recover. Doctors are not good at telling their patients that they will get better. But we've got to help you create the right circumstances for you to heal. You've been in a state of chronic stress and chronic inflammation and we need to get your cortisol levels down. What's your sleep like? We need to ensure that you're getting adequate sleep and rest, but I know you like exercise. Let's look at your exercise régime and see if we can gradually build your fitness. Your diet is really good, but knowing the importance of the gut biome [more on that later, reader], I suggest you have a daily dose of probiotic-rich yoghurt and we'll add some soluble fibre to supplement your diet. We need to deactivate your nervous system, which is in defensive mode. What are you like with meditation?

My partner wasn't working, but the advice from the GP was 'take time to heal, and we'll look at the question of timing for return to work next time'. As an occupational physician, specializing in rehabilitation and return to work, I could not fault her approach. Return to work was going to be part of the plan. It must be.

I was blown away by her approach. It was exactly how I would want to be treated by my doctor. She was very human. Her body language demonstrated empathy, the message that 'I can imagine what you must be going through', and compassion; so much caring and genuine sorrow at what she had been experiencing. There was no hierarchy in the approach, no feeling that the knowledge of the doctor was equated with power. This was a true partnership approach: the management plan was what 'we need' to do. It was a long appointment, which was charged accordingly, but we both left with a feeling of confidence, and indeed relief. There was a plan, a clear direction, an ability to control, and, most importantly, hope.

I was so focused on the outcome of the consultation and how impressed I was that I've only now realized something: the GP loved her job. She knew she was making a difference. From a GP's perspective, there was nothing unusual about the attendance—a patient with chronic illness coming for a medication review. I think that this is simply her consultation style, the service all her patients get. It did take more time, but the value-add from the additional service was invaluable. The patient's experience was one of great satisfaction. But so was the doctor's experience (Fig. 7.1).

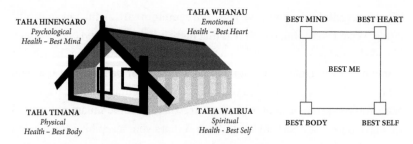

Fig. 7.1 Te whare tapa whā: the Māori model of health.

Te whare tapa whā in practice

I'm fortunate to work outside the healthcare system, without its time constraints. My client referrals are from employers or insurance companies. My assessments start by spending an hour to an hour and a half with a client. But prior to that I will usually have spent a similar amount of time going through all the GP and specialist records.

The first question I ask myself is 'What is the diagnosis?' That means reviewing the documented history, investigations, diagnosis and treatment, and treatment response. Almost by definition, since I see many complex cases, the treatment response has been poor, and people have not been able to return to work or get on with their lives. Statistically, we know that 10–20 per cent of diagnoses are wrong.[8] That is also my experience. So, I start my process by re-taking the history from the client, *really carefully*. I cannot state too strongly that people usually provide their own diagnosis; yet often assumptions have been made in the history provided (often to several different doctors) such that important clues have been missed. Yes, I do treat this as though I'm a medical detective!

You will also note that this stage of the process is very much what I've been trained to do: I apply the medical model. That has to be the first stage, the filtering process to identify any underlying pathology. If 10–20 per cent of the diagnoses are wrong, then one reason is that conditions change over time and diagnoses change over time. If I'm seeing someone who hasn't worked for 3 years and has been through the healthcare mill over that period, and often seen many different doctors, then the likelihood is that the diagnosis has changed over time. The original diagnosis might have been correct, but it has never been updated and the management process has not been aimed at the correct diagnosis.

My assessment process goes through all four domains of the cornerstones of the Māori model of health, te whare tapa whā: physical, psychological, family and emotional, and spiritual. Each part of the assessment gives me new insights into the person behind the symptoms. It is they who provide the answers, both in the diagnosis and also for what needs to happen. I'm going to describe each of these stages in more detail, but I just want to tackle the term 'spiritual' before I go any further. In 1985, Sir Mason Durie pointed out that the spiritual domain was missing from models of health for Māori, whereas in fact it was the single most important part of their health, and without it they were not considered to have health.[9] I use a very broad definition of spirituality, because it is my belief that we all have a belief in something beyond ourselves, in aspects of our life that bring purpose and meaning to it. These are the things that make it worth getting up in the morning. Chronic illness often means that these aspects of our life become neglected or are too hard. These elements may include religion, but in our increasingly secular world they may not. What is consistent is how we contribute to the lives of other people, how we add value, in our family, our work, and our communities. How we define our purpose, our reason for being. For this reason, I now refer to 'spiritual or existential health'. Existential being a philosophical concept that considers questions of what it means to be human, what brings meaning and purpose in our lives as individuals.

Sir Mason has also pointed out to me that the spiritual domain also relates to our interaction with our environment, the importance of our land, respect for our planet, and, for Māori, even their relationship with the stars and the cosmos.

Why don't doctors bring spirituality into the consultation? As discussed earlier, patients do see meaning and purpose as being an important part of a more holistic approach to healthcare. Yet it is still a subject many people find difficulty talking about in social settings. When I asked a friend if he had a belief system, he was quite taken aback and replied, 'What's it got to do with you?'

But surely along with the personal and intimate details of your life that you already discuss with your doctor, the conversation can include belief systems. My experience is that the majority of people I ask about their belief system in a clinical setting have no problem at all discussing it, and indeed welcome the in-depth conversation that ensues.

Nonetheless, a survey of doctors in Australia and New Zealand identified very clear reasons why doctors do find this difficult.[10] The main reason is that they confuse spirituality with religion and believe that patients won't want to be asked about it, or they feel uncomfortable themselves. They also worry about how their colleagues will perceive them. If spirituality is not traditionally seen as part of medicine, or if they are religious themselves, they fear that they will be thought to be preaching.

That's not what spirituality needs to look like in the consultation. I asked a big, burly, Southland farmer if he had a belief system. He said, 'Well, I was brought up Presbyterian, but I don't hold with any of that now. I tell you, if there was a God then none of the things I've seen in my life would have happened.'

He paused, and added, 'Don't get me wrong, I believe in something, I believe there's something bigger than us, that we're here for a purpose.'

I asked him what his purpose was. His chest puffed out, and he said, 'I'm the rock. I'm the head of the family. I'm the person everyone comes to for advice and support.' Then his shoulders slumped. 'At least I was. Haven't been for the last 2 years. Since the back injury. Now I just sit in the corner of the room and the family get on with things as if I wasn't there. I'm a spare part.'

There it was. That was what I needed to hear. He had lost his reason for being. Lost his purpose. In Māori, he had lost his mana. A complex word with layers of meaning, it encompasses respect and position in the wider family, the whānau, and the community, but it also means the spiritual power bestowed on a person by their ancestors. Here we had something we could work with: a huge motivation for him to participate in the programme to help him move forward with his life and regain his purpose and role in his family.

The authors of the research on attitudes of doctors discussing spirituality called for a model of practice they described as 'biopsychosocial–spiritual',[11] in other words, including the four domains of the Māori model of health.[12] They noted that, increasingly, spirituality in medicine is being taught at medical school, and they expressed hope it will increasingly come into medical practice. They included a quote from one of the doctors who participated in the study:

> My understanding, because I believe in holistic care, is that if I need to talk about sexuality, I should talk about sexuality. If I need to talk about faith, I should talk about faith. If I need to talk about bowels, I should talk about bowels ... Some people would say that in every initial consultation a question about people's sexuality ... is standard. Well—that's not what I've done either.[13]

The researchers commented, 'Human sexuality is very important to patients, even during sickness, but discussion causes discomfort for doctors and is not routinely included in medical consultations. Ditto spirituality. However, there will be occasions when to ignore the spiritual dimension is to ignore one of the most important contributions to patient distress, or one of the most important coping mechanisms available to them.'[14]

I'm sure you know me well enough by now to know that I do include discussion about sexuality in my assessments (introduced sensitively, of course). I don't find it uncomfortable, and neither do my clients. I strongly suspect the discomfort felt by doctors is because they (falsely) consider their patients will be uncomfortable to be asked. There is research available which identifies more of the reasons. In a survey of 813 doctors, 90 per cent considered that addressing sexuality should be part of the holistic care of patients. However, almost all of them, 94 per cent, didn't do it.[15] The main reason they gave was inadequate training. Inevitably, the conclusion was that more training is needed.

The second stage of my process is communication. With the client's consent, I share the assessment report (which is long and detailed) with their GP, specialists, and allied health professionals. Then I seek their input, including by telephone discussion. It's really important to both me and the client that I've taken into account the views of their treating doctor, and especially have obtained their buy-in to the process. These conversations have to be sensitive ones, because I may have concluded that the diagnosis was incorrect. However, my report contains my reasoning as to why that is the case. One common reason I find the diagnosis to be incorrect is that a chronic pain disorder affecting one region (a shoulder, for instance) is often misdiagnosed as a shoulder pathological condition, which then doesn't respond to surgery. The central mediation of pain in chronic pain syndromes has not yet been fully integrated into medical education. Only last week a specialist asked me, 'Could you explain what a central sensitization disorder is, please?'

The third stage is the planning stage. Taking about an hour, I work through each of the four domains with the client and we actively, together, look for ways forward to address the issues identified. Some of them may be medical, and will have been discussed with the relevant doctor (for instance, medication changes), but most will be in terms of steps the person can take to gain control of their own circumstances and symptoms. By the time we've worked through the four domains, we've got a plan, and also clarity as to whether other health professional input is required: psychologist, physiotherapist, or occupational therapist. If we need to look at alternative employment, then we may also include a vocational consultant to look at transferable skills or training needs. The plan is written up in the first person, as 'My Life and Health Integration Plan'. Where possible I use quotes, the exact description the person has described. Describing the plan as 'I will ...' increases ownership and empowerment because it places the responsibility for success on the individual. Too often in rehabilitation programmes the client is told what to do and how to do it, but there is little buy-in. The client feels the programme is being done *to* them, not for and *with* them.

I call it a Life and Health Integration Plan, because it does what it says on the tin—it integrates the four domains of health into every part of the client's life. As they work through the process, they realize the power of the integration: to have physical health improves psychological health, which impacts the quality of relationships, and all are driven by spiritual health, the growing realization of what brings meaning and purpose in their lives. This in turn provides the motivation to continue to make positive choices and embed them as habits and routines. Habits trump willpower every day!

Gayle's experience of the positive medicine process
Being chronically ill or in pain progressively changes all aspects of one's life. Many of the changes are so gradual that it is easy to forget what it is like to be yourself, and genuinely healthy. For me, in part because of the nature of the illness itself, and in part because of the protracted time that lapsed, I made many changes to my behaviour that I don't readily identify with as myself. I changed the ways in which I engaged with others. I stopped taking part in all of the activities I enjoyed doing most. I put things off, hoping for a day when things were better, but when those days came I had so many things that needed my attention that little to nothing was done that was on my 'want to' list. I ended up only engaging in the 'have to' and activities that helped me to cope on the bad days, rather than spending time doing things that bring me joy, satisfaction, and fulfilment. In many ways, this led me to neglect my sense of well-being, and reduced the amount of restorative and healing practices as well as significantly reducing my overall quality of life.

The process that David has created as a health facilitation plan engages all aspects of oneself. It addresses the lifestyle behaviours that contribute to poorer health and replaces them with habits that are restorative and can progress into a lifestyle that will maintain better health outcomes. The acknowledgement of what I had forgotten in myself and the understanding of the importance of incrementally including small changes to align my behaviour with how I see myself as a person was, for me, fundamental to progressing from the mindset of a chronically ill person to a person with a sense of fulfilment who considers the future with optimism.

Integrating the plan into my life was easy. While I was guided through the process, the plan was a result of my own reflection and my own decisions.

One can get advice and integrate it if it feels right, but I have always felt that we fundamentally know what we need (even if we don't want to admit it to ourselves) and what we need to do for ourselves, just as much as we know what we enjoy doing. At the end of the day, it is me who has to heal me. I may get help from many avenues of medical and wellbeing practices, but I still have to do the work myself and continue taking care of myself for as long as I am alive.

My medical and counselling team were all contacted and approached during the process of developing the plan and continued communicating as required as I worked through the steps. To me, it is fundamental that everyone is understanding of the process. Some of the steps in the recovery process are harder to climb than others, and support and understanding are essential if one is able to create and maintain the behaviour changes. I also feel that my ongoing illness was not a straightforward one. I think that my medical team were grateful for the opportunity to have the support of the whole team to share the responsibility of assisting me in my recovery.

I am so grateful for how much progress I have made with my health and my wellbeing in the short time I have been working with this process. Many of my physiological limitations still exist, but I have better tools to manage them, a better understanding of how to continue living despite them, and, most importantly, an improved sense of purpose with which to make decisions in order to continue leading a fulfilling life. And I have the motivation and energy to continue to work on incrementally making changes to carry on improving.

Clearly, the kind of complex cases I'm describing involve people at the tertiary phase of dis-ease, when injury, disease, or illness has already occurred. But the process works just as effectively, and perhaps in a more straightforward way, at the primary prevention level, before any issues have developed; and at a secondary stage, when the person is in a state of dis-ease but illness and disease haven't yet occurred. This often means that the person feels out of control of their life and destiny, and knows they are stressed, but hasn't worked out what they need to do about it.

Considering the tiers of Maslow's hierarchy of needs, the issue could be occurring at any level of the hierarchy, but the natural human motivation is the drive to become the best we can be in the circumstances. The circumstances may be financial, work related, or relationship or family related. Often it is a combination of the three. By putting in place a Life and Health Integration Plan, the person is placed in the best position to take control of their circumstances.

The plan will include strategies and resources, and may include input from specific professionals to further develop and empower the person.

Over the next four chapters, we will look at some specifics to see how the whole comes together as a consolidated plan. The aim is to improve function and quality of life, and therefore to improve people's happiness and sense of fulfilment in life.

Using a positive psychology model, I see the ultimate goal as being flourishing, or, using Maslow's motivational model, as self-actualization. I contacted Martin Seligman to ask if he thought that flourishing was the modern equivalent of self-actualization. His response was that he felt that it was entirely possible to achieve flourishing without meeting all the tiers of Maslow's model, and that the concept of flourishing was more to do with our interaction with other people than self-actualization, which is focused on the individual. In all honesty, I'm not sure I agree with him. Maslow made clear that the tiers were not fixed, and Maslow very much described self-actualized people in terms of their positive relations with others. I think flourishing is equivalent to self-actualization and is the natural progression from Maslow's 1943 model.

Positive medicine integrates the medical model with the Māori model of health, Maslow's model of motivation, and the concept of flourishing in Martin Seligman's wellbeing theory, to help people attain positive health.

8

Physical Health—Te Taha Tinana

In the Māori model of health, te whare tapa whā, Sir Mason Durie points out that one of the four cornerstones, physical health, is the focus of Western medicine. Here the search for disease is predominant and here too any attempts at health promotion are made. But Sir Mason points out that, for Māori, there are many traditions and practices that support the health of the body, including the sacredness of the preparation of food and its deliberate separation from bodily functions such as toileting. Maslow saw this bottom tier of his model as being the bedrock, the foundation: the physiological needs of the person, without which even survival is in question. He saw the physiological function of the body as having primacy above all others. He knew the body to be a sophisticated system of incredibly refined feedback loops and, further, that the body will do anything to try to keep its physiology within finely tuned parameters. He knew this to be called homeostasis.

As Martin Seligman said to me, to flourish doesn't mean that all tiers of Maslow's hierarchy are fulfilled. Maslow himself said this, but he also said, 'A person who is lacking food, safety, love, and esteem would probably hunger for food more strongly than for anything else.' Seligman's wellbeing theory, with its five components of positive emotion, engagement, relationships, meaning, and achievement (PERMA) lacks a clear physical component. Subsequent positive psychologists have added a sixth component, vitality. In true positive psychology style, the word conjures up a vision of positivity and optimism. To have vitality means the body is fully functioning, active, truly alive! So, let's take that into the mix. It seems a very good goal for us to aim for.

Vitality and ageing

'Vitality' is not a word I would have used to describe myself back in 2003, when I had my heart attack. At the age of 42 I had let myself go. I was physically unfit, overweight, probably drinking too much. I had poor sleep, stressful work, poor

Positive Medicine. David Beaumont, Oxford University Press. © Oxford University Press 2021.
DOI: 10.1093/oso/9780192845184.003.0009

work–life balance (although I will debunk that expression in Chapter 9), and all the responsibilities of a young family.

My wife, during my recovery, had observed, 'You look like an old man' and that's how I felt. I definitely looked after my physical health better after that scare, but to be honest, I was a bit half-hearted. However, my 50th birthday felt a bit of a shock to me. Fifty? *Really?* I absolutely didn't feel 50. In my mind, and in my vision of myself, I felt 32. And that stuck. If anyone asks me now how old I am, without hesitation I reply 32.

It turns out that there is science behind this approach. Before I explain the science, I'll give you a further example to illustrate that age is a frame of mind. My brother-in-law came over to New Zealand from the UK. He's the same age as me, and had just been diagnosed with type 2 diabetes. I was quite shocked to see how much he had aged since I had last seen him. He had been told he had to lose weight, to get rid of that paunch. The first day, he and I went for a walk along the lakeside. I struggled to walk as slowly as him. He was taking slow, deliberate steps and was hunched over.

I asked, 'Paul, how old do you feel?'

Without hesitation, he said, 'Seventy.'

Yep, that's exactly how old he looked, too. I talked to him about the science behind thought and ageing, and we agreed that the timing could not be better for him to take some control of his health. Over the course of the next month, Paul started walking or cycling every day. His shape changed, his demeanour changed, he walked faster, stood more upright, and his weight dropped. By the time he left New Zealand to return home, he looked 20 years younger.

Intriguingly, 2 years before that, his father, my then-father-in-law, had done exactly the same thing. Brian is a man with a medical history as long as your arm, and when he arrived in New Zealand, he looked ... well, I think I would offend him if I said how old he looked. But it doesn't matter, because after 3 months of doing my gardening every day, he was brown as a berry, leaner, faster, grinning. We went to visit a friend whose house had a swimming pool. My mate came into the house and said, 'David, quick, come outside, you've got to see this!'

There was Brian, showing off to the kids, doing handstands underwater in the pool!

The science behind the concept that 'you're only as old as you feel' began in 1979, when a psychologist took a group of men in their 70s from a nursing home environment to take part in an experiment. They were placed in a time warp situation; the world as it had been 20 years earlier. If our environment affects our health, then could a change of environment improve health?

The study participants were played music from 1959, were given newspapers from that year, and were told to behave as though they were 20 years younger. There were even photos of them from 20 years before.

Just a week later, reported the study's author, Professor Ellen Langer, the men showed improvements in many areas of function: 'physical strength, manual dexterity, gait, posture, perception, memory, cognition, taste sensitivity, hearing and vision.'[1] One reason may be the placebo effect, and the power of belief. The study participants were told that the intention of the study was that they would feel as they did 20 years earlier. They believed, and it happened.

In 1984, the science behind ageing and anti-ageing suddenly got much more, well, *scientific*, with the discovery by Professor Elizabeth Blackburn (and her PhD student Carol Greider) of the enzyme telomerase, for which they were awarded the Nobel Prize in Physiology or Medicine in 2009. Telomerase, Blackburn discovered, looks after our telomeres. Telomeres are the structures that protect our DNA strands. They are best pictured as the plastic caps that cover the tips of shoelaces to stop them fraying. It turns out that at each cell replication our DNA can be damaged, with the tips of the strands being particularly vulnerable. Repair happens all the time, and it is the telomerase that repairs the strands to allow the cell to keep on reproducing. But once the telomeres have broken down, that's it, the protection for the end of the strand has gone. The DNA frays, just as a shoelace does once the tip has broken, and the cell dies because it can no longer divide and replicate.

Blackburn's research has focused on the effects of stress on ageing and disease. Chronic stress leads to reduced telomerase function in the body, which in turn leads to premature cell ageing and disease.

But it turns out we have choices. We can take control of our life and health. In her book *The Telomere Effect: A Revolutionary Approach to Living Younger, Healthier, Longer*, Blackburn explains:

> Your telomeres, it turns out, are listening to you. They absorb the instructions you give them. The way you live can, in effect, tell your telomeres to speed up the process of cellular ageing. But it can also do the opposite. The foods you eat, your response to emotional challenges, the amount of exercise you get, whether you were exposed to childhood stress, and even the level of trust and safety in your neighbourhood—all of these factors and more appear to influence your telomeres and can prevent premature ageing at the cellular level. In short, one of the keys to a long healthspan is simply doing your part to foster healthy cell renewal.[2]

Healthspan is a concept that is well described. Its opposite is known as *diseasespan*, defined as the length of time we spend living our lives in disease, rather than health. Clearly, the ideal is to live as high a proportion of our lives in health as possible, and then simply drop off our proverbial perch. The alternative is premature disease and morbidity and living out our remaining years in pain and disability.

Increasingly, the evidence is that we can influence that with our lifestyle choices.

Don't get me wrong. I have spent the last 6 years on a journey of self-discovery and search for optimum health for myself. It has been easy to define what I want from optimum health, because I have experienced the opposite: illness, disease, disability, chronic pain, and depression (more on this in Chapter 9). On my journey, I have read many, many books from the health and wellbeing section in bookshops.

Oh my goodness, the wealth of science and cutting-edge thinking and thought leadership I have discovered there! Can I be honest, and say that in my years as a traditional doctor I would never have ventured into that part of the bookshop. I didn't need to, of course, because I had my medical training. What it has done for me is to open my eyes to a completely different world, which is just as much science as medical science (and often way beyond the concepts of medical science). But I'm not reading these books alone. Many, many people are devouring these books and developing a level of knowledge that may not be shared by their doctors.

The conclusions about what constitutes optimum health and wellbeing will come as no surprise to the readers of these books, and they are also completely intuitive to all of us. Now, I have discovered, we have the science behind it too.

The answer lies in exercise and activity, good nutrition, restorative sleep, stretching our muscles and joints, breathing and mindfulness meditation practices, dealing with our demons (more on that in Chapter 9), and therefore dealing with our bad habits. (Addictive behaviours such as smoking and drinking are intimately linked to our demons.) These are the habits that lead on to what Machteld Huber, Martin Seligman, and others have called positive health. So, let's call them 'the life habits of positive health'.

There are literally thousands of books on the subject of healthy lifestyle, and mountains of research to provide the science. My intention in this book is not to deal with the what, but rather the how and the why. In Simon Sinek style, we should start with *why*, and the how and the what will flow on naturally. The 'why' for me is that (for the most part) doctors are not currently anywhere to be seen in health and wellbeing. Yet they could be making an enormous difference to the lives and health of their patients. The 'how' is to operationalize whole-person models of health, such as the Māori model of health, into models of practice for doctors; empowering patients to take control of their life and develop the habits of positive health by practising positive medicine.

Interestingly, it turns out that the 'what' is pretty much the same at a primary, secondary, and tertiary level of prevention. What do you do if you're young and healthy and stay like that? You develop the habits of positive health. What do you do if you've already got illness or disease? You develop the habits of positive health. I would suggest you buy a book. One I would recommend that has the science attached is Elizabeth Blackburn's *The Telomere Effect*.[3]

The other book you should read is by Dr David Sinclair: *Lifespan: Why We Age – and Why We Don't Have To*. David Sinclair describes the advances created by 'the new science of ageing'.[4] He explains the evolutionary mechanisms for ageing, and how our bodies interact with our environment. The answer? Epigenetics—the science of gene expression.

From the time that the human genome was first mapped, in 2004, we understood the blueprint for human life. Or we thought we did. A new science was growing—one that caused David Sinclair to say 'Our genes are not our destiny'.

There's a glaring problem with seeing our DNA as being what shapes us. That is that every cell in our bodies contains the same DNA. And yet we have thousands of different types of cells: skin cells, heart cells, brain cells. They look and function completely differently. Why? Because the genes that are made up of DNA have been turned on or off, by the process of epigenetics.

Our epigenome is how we interact with our world, our environment. It's what causes genes to be expressed or repressed.

If all the DNA in a single human cell were unwound, it would stretch nearly 2 metres. But, double-stranded DNA is tightly woven around proteins called histones, which form multiple spools called chromatins. The shape of these spools changes constantly, causing sites on our genes to be exposed or hidden. It is the shape of our DNA, and whether certain molecules (known as acetyl and methyl groups) are bound to the DNA, that determines which proteins our DNA causes to be manufactured.

There are multiple mechanisms by which we age. All of them are controlled by epigenetics. And how our genes are expressed is impacted by how we interact with our environment. Identical twins have exactly the same DNA. As babies, they look identical. The older they get, the more their appearance differs. This is because they have a different experience of life, and therefore different gene expression.

Nature or nurture? Genes or environment? Epigenetics now explains this centuries-old dilemma. Our genes are the blueprint, our genotype; but how we turn out, our phenotype (our body shape, our ageing, even our diseases), is determined by how we intact with our environment, through the mechanisms of epigenetics.

How do we interact with our environment? Through our exposures (to the purity of the air we breathe, ultraviolet light in sunlight, and the food we take into our bodies), our experience of life (how we live our lives, our activities, exercise, and sleep), and what we believe about our experiences. There are fast and slow epigenetic mechanisms. Negative emotions or positive emotions can turn genes on or off in a matter of minutes.

Now we have a mechanism to explain why different life experiences cause different life courses—differences in health and disease, and length of life. Yes, David Sinclair agrees with Elizabeth Blackburn, that she is correct in identifying telomere length as being one of the determinants of ageing and death (and he quotes her research). He also agrees that our experience of life, and the habits of positive health she describes, impact the length of telomeres, and therefore longevity. The mechanism is by production of the enzyme which protects telomere length, telomerase. The amount of telomerase varies with our life experience. Telomerase is a protein, and the production of that protein in relation to our environment is determined by ... epigenetics.

If every protein in our bodies is produced as a response to epigenetic mechanisms, in relation to our interactions with our environment, our life, and our world, then surely epigenetics answers everything? Health, disease, and lifespan?

Sir Harry Burns believes that epigenetics may answer, at least in part, the Glasgow effect—why the people of Glasgow experience disproportionately bad health.

Surely epigenetics explains the health gradient that Sir Michael Marmot identified in relation to the social determinants of health?

I asked the director of the Dunedin Study, Professor Richie Poulton, whether epigenetic mechanisms explained the differences in health identified in people having different life experiences. He said, 'No. Epigenetics provides a mechanism for nature and nurture to interact.'

About how our life unfolds, David Sinclair says:

The pianist that makes this happen is the epigenome. By the process of revealing our DNA or bundling it up in tight protein packages, and by making genes with chemical tags called methyls and acetyls composed of carbon, oxygen, and hydrogen, the epigenome uses our genome to make the music of our lives.

Let's explore tertiary prevention further. If you've had a heart attack, then there is clear evidence, from the principles of cardiac rehabilitation, that to develop the habits of positive health reduces your risk of further heart events and mortality. The same with respiratory disease, and also with arthritis and musculo-skeletal conditions. What's the treatment for type 2 diabetes? There are many drugs, such as metformin, that are used to try to control the effects of insulin resistance in type 2 diabetes. However, somewhat startlingly, the evidence is that many cases of type 2 diabetes can be successfully treated, and the person can return to a normal weight, normal blood sugar, and physiological homeostasis, by developing the habits of positive health.

There's a slight challenge in what I'm going to say next, because it is an area of great sensitivity for people with medically unexplained symptoms.

There is abundant evidence that there are two modalities of management that have positive benefits for people with medically unexplained symptoms. The evidence is that it does not matter whether you have chronic fatigue (CFS/ME), fibromyalgia, chronic pain in other regions, or irritable bowel syndrome; both modalities are likely to benefit you.

Those two modalities are graded exercise therapy and cognitive behavioural therapy (CBT, combined with treating depression, if depression is present). But many people with medically unexplained symptoms do not like to be confronted with this evidence, often because they feel it's so simple that it must be affirming the concept that 'it's all in the mind'. But that's the point! This is all simple, as the best solutions usually are. There is no difference whether you have an illness such as a medically unexplained symptom, a disease like diabetes or cancer, a disease predisposition such as obesity, or chronic pain after an injury—the answer is to develop the habits of positive health!

I said earlier that Matt had pointed out to me that positive medicine was a great concept, even if the only person it helped was me. So, the last 6 years have been spent on the journey of developing the habits of positive health through my own practice of positive medicine on the patient I know best of all—me!

My journey back to health

First things first, in acknowledgement of the medical model and the fact that I am at the tertiary end of the prevention spectrum (since I have had a heart attack, hip osteoarthritis, chronic pain and disability, and depression), it is very important that I am registered with a doctor and see him for 6-monthly reviews and blood tests. (I should add that many doctors are so poor at looking after their own health that they don't even have a doctor.) I'm also very good at taking my medication. My blood pressure, cholesterol, and other parameters are well in the normal, homeostatic range. The habits of positive health are so interlinked that it's hard to separate them out.

The first thing I tackled was being overweight. The answer was a combination of exercise, nutritional changes, and mindfulness meditation (to reduce cortisol, which is an obesogenic hormone—that is, it promotes obesity). At the start this was hard, because walking aggravated the pain from my hip osteoarthritis, but I discovered that cycling didn't. Even better was aquajogging, which is basically jogging in the deep end of the swimming pool, wearing a floatation belt. Once I had had first one, then the other hip joint replaced with metal and ceramic prosthetic hips, I was truly bionic, and there was no holding me back. I now rotate my exercise routine between walking, swimming, cycling, and gym work. And yoga. Once my hips were replaced, I realized just how stiff I had become. My hip flexors were so tight I couldn't stand up straight. I was walking with my bum sticking out, a duck walk!

That took some correcting, but with physiotherapy and stretch class I was amazed how much difference it made. And, bonus, the long-standing low-back pain I had suffered completely disappeared, and never came back. The discovery of yoga has been amazing. Always stiff-jointed, and getting worse with age, I would never have thought I would be able to get into the positions I have. Yoga has the additional benefit of teaching breathing techniques and incorporating meditation modalities.

In order to address weight loss, I also carefully researched nutrition. It's a minefield, isn't it? Seems to change week by week.

An internationally recognized guru on the science behind nutrition and diet is Dr Michael Mosley, a UK doctor, producer, and BBC TV presenter. Credited with popularizing the 5:2 diet after describing his own journey of regaining health after a diagnosis of type 2 diabetes, he has since devised his own evidence-based diets, including the Blood Sugar Diet and more recently The Fast800 diet.[5] I like his approach and the research backing, and also the human evolutionary context. Our ancestors were not designed to have three meals a day, but their bodies were geared up to periods of fasting—burning stored fats (as fatty acids and ketones) rather than relying on rapidly available sources such as glucose and other sugars. His work also resonated with me after reading the work of Professor Grant Schofield here in New Zealand, whose books *What the*

Fat? and *What the Fast?* promote a healthy fat, Mediterranean diet, with low carbohydrates and intermittent fasting.[6]

It's not surprising that the research is confusing, and that people find they yoyo with dieting (weight goes up and down with diet, but with a gradual trend upwards!). What Michael Mosley concludes is that whether your diet is high fat–high carb, low fat–low carb, high protein–low carb, paleo, and so on, diets generally all work initially, and often if you stick at them. The key is how sustainable the diet is. His three steps to successful weight loss are:

- Personalize the diet to you.
- Lose weight and reprogram your body.
- Learn for life.

For me, there were some key things that worked and that I've stuck at and learned for life. First, bread *really* doesn't suit me. Oh, the relief from bloating that I gained when I stopped bread! And beer as well. Second, both Michael Mosley and Grant Schofield introduced me to the notion that 'breakfast should be the main meal of the day' is a complete myth!

Breakfast is the one meal I thought I could never go without. I used to eat cereal with hidden sugars for breakfast and find I was hungry 2 hours later and needing a mid-morning snack. I've reprogrammed my body to burn fats and ketones (as it is designed to do). Now I try to have at least a 12-hour overnight fast (which switches the body from carbohydrates to ketones). On many days I have a 16-hour fast, only having calories in the remaining 8 hours (eating low-carbohydrate, higher-protein foods, and healthy fats like olive oil and avocado). I usually only eat two meals per day, with snacks of fresh fruit and dried fruit and nuts between. The 13.5 kg (30 pounds) I lost initially I've largely kept off, with minor fluctuations. I'm not on a diet, but I have a nutritional habit as part of my habits of positive health.

The importance of sleep as part of the picture cannot be overstated. There's a good collection of the science behind sleep at healthline.com, backing up the following ten points:

- Poor sleep increases the risk of obesity.
- Good sleepers produce lower levels of obesogenic hormones (those that promote fat storage).
- Good sleep promotes brain function: cognition, concentration, productivity, and performance.
- Good sleep promotes activity and exercise performance.

- Poor sleep is a risk factor for heart disease and stroke.
- Sleep affects glucose metabolism and therefore the risk of diabetes.
- Depression results in poor sleep, but poor sleep also increases the risk of depression.
- Sleep improves immune function. Poor sleep decreases immunity.
- Poor sleep increases inflammatory markers, and aggravates chronic inflammatory conditions (such as inflammatory bowel disease).
- Disturbed sleep affects our ability to pick up social and emotional cues and affects social interactions.

I try to ensure I have 7–8 hours of sleep per night. How do I feel? Better than I've felt for decades. How old do I feel? Thirty-two. Fitter, more active, more flexible, with more energy.

But physical health is only a quarter of the picture. There are three other cornerstones to my health. I'll cover those in the following chapters.

9

Psychological Health—
Te Taha Hinengaro

As we saw in Chapter 6, in his exposition of the Māori model of health, Sir Mason Durie explained that thoughts and feelings are an integral part of health for Māori. He pointed out that Māori traditional thinking is holistic, whereas traditional Western medical thinking is analytical. He noted that to integrate psychological health into medicine has been challenging and tortuous: '[E]ven now the concept often rests uneasily alongside a wealth of knowledge derived from physical sciences.'[1]

Abraham Maslow saw this next tier of the pyramid, safety needs, being only just above the physiological needs. Once a person had their basic needs met and were no longer hungry, then the greatest desire is to feel safe. At its most extreme form, the fear or threat of danger and therefore the desire for safety may become all-consuming, to the exclusion of everything else. If this is true for adults, then this becomes far more the case for children, who are vulnerable and dependent. Maslow spends a good deal of time considering the effects of adverse childhood experiences. He paints a bleak picture, describing how terrifying these experiences must be to children; the feelings of rejection, of terror, and of lack of safety. In this fear he sees the roots of adult illness, particularly psychological illness.

For Martin Seligman, to achieve flourishing is to experience positive emotions. This is the aim, too, of positive psychology. (It's what the P of PERMA, in the wellbeing model, stands for.) Seligman pulled back from his original idea that happiness was the key goal of wellbeing, but nevertheless, the love and happiness end of the spectrum remains the goal of wellbeing.

If there is a truth for us all, the Dalai Lama says that it is in the contrast between happiness and suffering. He says, 'From the moment of birth, every human being wants happiness and does not want suffering ... Therefore it is important to discover what will bring about the greatest degree of happiness.' His answer? That it lies in love and compassion, for others as much as for ourselves.[2]

Positive Medicine. David Beaumont, Oxford University Press. © Oxford University Press 2021.
DOI: 10.1093/oso/9780192845184.003.0010

The storms of life

New Zealand has a problem, and we haven't been addressing it. Every year, 20,000 people in New Zealand attempt suicide and 500 people die by suicide (that's in a country of 5 million people). Ours is among the worst rates of youth suicide in the 37 countries in the Organization for Economic Cooperation and Development (OECD). There's another big problem, and that is mental health in the workplace. Here's a strange thing; if it's a problem, why do we call it 'mental health'? It sounds as though it should be a positive concept, but it's actually a term used to represent mental *ill* health.

Mental health in the workplace represents the effects of bullying and harassment and discrimination. We're obscuring the picture by mixing up terms. We would not refer to 'physical health' as a negative concept. I suspect it is related to regarding anything with the word *mental* in it as having a negative context, which is part of the stigma that surrounds mental ill health and addiction. (Addictive behaviour is often seen in, at best, a judgement context, or at worst, is criminalized.) Yet mental ill health affects the majority of us.

In the 2018 Government Inquiry into Mental Health and Addiction, the problem was defined (spanning 'the full spectrum from mental distress to full psychiatric illness'), and solutions were recommended.[3] The Inquiry found that, every year, one in five New Zealanders experience mental illness or significant mental distress. Between 50 and 80 per cent will experience such conditions or addiction, or both, at some point in their lives. That's most of us.

The New Zealand comedian Mike King campaigns for better mental health in New Zealand. At first, he was strongly criticized for going around schools and talking about youth suicide. Mike believes we have to be able to talk about it, let it be OK to discuss, and thus make it easy for people to seek help. I recently attended a conference where he spoke. He started by asking the audience how many of us had experienced suicidal thoughts at some time in our lives: almost all of the audience put their hands up.

The annual cost of mental ill health in New Zealand is thought to be $12 billion, or 5 per cent of gross domestic product.

The Inquiry saw the roots of the problem as being in the social determinants of health, particularly poverty, and the lack of an integrated response up to now. What did the people they interviewed want?

> [A] call for wellbeing and community solutions—for help through the storms of life, to be seen as a whole person, not a diagnosis, and to be encouraged and supported to heal and restore one's sense of self.[4]

People were asking for help to become empowered, to be able to adapt and self-manage in the face of life's challenges—the new definition of health. The solutions the Inquiry team recommended were comprehensive, but they stressed the need for them to be integrated, to be community and family orientated, and to address the social determinants of health. They pointed out that primary care reforms and new models of care had previously been recommended, but not put in place. But even in the face of a need for a wellbeing approach, the role they saw for primary care, and general practice particularly, was very much a treatment-based approach.

Six months after the publication of the review, the New Zealand government produced its first 'Wellbeing Budget', focused on measures to address inequity and the social determinants of health, to improve the wellbeing of the population. It put 'Taking our mental health seriously' to the forefront.[5]

In my assessments of this psychological cornerstone of our health, I look for evidence of depression, anxiety, or other forms of mental ill health or distress. Then I go on to measures of happiness and quality of life. But I also explore the history for the presence of stressors, recent or distant, including childhood. There is a school of thought that sees all emotions as being subsets of only two basic emotions: love and fear. Pain is an emotional response and at its root lies fear. As we have already seen, the presence of stressors, which include physical or psychological trauma, and particularly adverse childhood experiences is a marker or risk factor for the development of chronic pain.

Part of the solution may lie in dealing with that trauma and reducing the level of fear. One way to remove the emotional interpretation of pain is to turn it into something measurable and objective. Traditionally, this is measured by asking the person to rate their pain on a scale of 1–10, where 10 is the worst pain imaginable. Because this is necessarily subjective, it automatically includes an emotional component. People will often score their pain to me at levels of 8, 9, or 10. In chronic pain syndromes, because the pain is centrally mediated and the brain over-sensitized, even though the person has been asked to rate the pain on a scale up to ten, they will often say, '12' or '20' to reflect just how horrible their pain is.

A few years ago, I was presenting at the New Zealand Pain Society conference. It was just before my second hip replacement, and I was in constant pain. One of the speakers presented on a technique to utilize meditation for pain management. As I listened to the technique, I was fascinated, so I decided to try it while he was presenting. (Yes, I did miss the rest of his talk!)

Try it for yourself. Most people have aches and pains to some degree, somewhere, or you may have a painful condition or suffer from chronic pain. First, rate the pain on how severe it is (1–10). Then, rate it again on scales that are not traditionally applied to pain, but seem more objective. What *speed* is your pain (slow–fast, 1–10). What *density* is your pain? (diffuse–very dense, 1–10). What *temperature* is your pain? (cold–hot, 1–10). Now, close your eyes, take some deep, slow breaths, in and out. Become aware of your surroundings, the feel of your thighs on the seat, your feet on the floor. Then listen, what can you hear? (Wherever I am, indoors or outside, even in the city, I can always hear a bird singing!)

Now, pay attention to your breath. Don't control it, just let it flow in and out, but feel it flow in and out of your nostrils. OK, now open your eyes, rate the speed, density, and temperature of your pain again. What did you find?

I was astounded at the degree of pain reduction in the space of 5 minutes.

Pain is a response to fear. It's the brain going into defensive mode because it is afraid of a threat (real or perceived). Making the pain more objective starts to take the emotional component, the fear, out of it. But there's an extension to this—not just removing the emotion, but replacing it with the opposite of fear, love. When Brian, my client in Chapter 5 with chronic pain in his arm, got caught up in winning at poker, doing something he loved, he got so caught up in a state of flow that his pain completely left him for the duration, and for hours afterwards!

My own experience with mental ill health started with chronic pain—oh, and throw marital breakdown into the mix. Relationship breakdown is one of life's challenges and sadly one that is very common. In fact, most of us will experience a relationship breakdown, with or without marriage. They're never easy. As I have come to know myself better, including through therapy, I have realized that my maladaptive strategies (the ways of coping that are not serving me well) include ruminating and catastrophizing. Ruminating is going through my take on what is happening over and over and over and over again. Catastrophizing fits really well with ruminating—but in a bad way! It means seeing what could go wrong, and imaging that it does. Then realizing that it could be even worse than that, and picturing what *that* would be like, until you see it as a catastrophe that will inevitably happen. What a great way to provoke fear!

Dealing with chronic pain in my hips meant that my sleep was disturbed. I just couldn't get comfortable. (Night pain in hip osteoarthritis is very common.) I was surviving on 3 or 4 hours of sleep a night, but there were those horrible, horrible nights when I couldn't sleep at all. Being tired and not sleeping makes you emotional, and I was crying most days; in taxis, on planes. Just quietly; no one knew. Then came the suicidal thoughts. They were very bleak. I know what it means when people talk about 'the dark night of the soul'.[6] Every time they came, I thought about my children. Rationally, I knew I wouldn't do anything. Eventually (I know, why did it take me so long?) I went to see my GP. He was amazing. Told me that he understood what I must be feeling, showing great empathy and compassion.

He said, 'You're depressed. We need to start you on antidepressants, get you to a psychologist, and decide what we're going to do about work.'

We agreed that because of the type of work I do as a doctor, which is more assessment and advisory than prescribing and operating, and the importance of work to me, that I could carry on working. But he said I had to halve my working hours and he would monitor the situation on a weekly basis. He warned me that antidepressants take 2 weeks to kick in, before I would feel any difference. He also reassured me I was going to recover.

I woke on the morning of the 15th day. I vividly recall shaving, looking in the mirror. Something was different. I looked different. My image in the mirror was clearer. I noticed that the sun was streaming into the bathroom. The mists were clearing.

My first emotion, interestingly, was anger. I was initially very angry that no one had told me I was depressed! It was really, really obvious. But not to me, and not as I was going through it. What I learned later was that anger was good. It was much, much better than the despondency I had been feeling, and was a step on the way to better and better emotions. From that time, I extolled the virtue of antidepressants! As I've researched the evidence, the jury really is still out as to how much effect they do have, and probably not much, or no better than placebo. On the other hand, I had just been given a clear diagnosis, a good prognosis, and had been treated with empathy and compassion—all the hallmarks of success for a placebo. I was told it would take 2 weeks to take effect and it took 14 days!

In retrospect, I think I was given a large, and very effective dose of 'the drug, doctor'.

For the second time in my life, I found myself in counselling with a psychologist. This time I was told the modality of talking therapy I would receive, called ACT or acceptance and commitment therapy. It was explained to me that I was in a state of fear, and that I would be trained in the techniques to overcome it, to help me understand how my way of dealing with my life challenges was leading to FEAR:

Fusion with my thoughts. Oh yes, all that ruminating!

Evaluation of my experience. Yep, that was the catastrophizing.

Avoidance. I would have done anything to get out of the situation.

Reason-giving. Trust me, in my hours of ruminating, I thought up lots of reasons.

In place of FEAR, I was taught how to ACT:

Accept the situation and be present in the moment.

Choose a valued direction. I had to define my values and find my purpose.

Take action. I developed an action plan.

One of the key components of the modality is mindfulness meditation. This is when I was first taught the technique that I regard as a fundamental part of my daily routine. The description I gave earlier for a technique in chronic pain was a very basic description, but actually the point is that it is simple to learn, and like everything else in life, you get better with practice.

In a state of mindful breathing, thoughts will come and go, but the idea is that you accept them, don't try to do anything about them, don't judge them, but let them drift away and be replaced by other thoughts. Also, be aware of the power of the moment. In this particular moment, here and now, is what I am fearing happening? No! I might be still worrying that it will happen, but it isn't actually occurring here and now.

Our minds are very good at going over the events of the past, and worrying about the future. To bring our awareness into the peace of the present moment is a powerful tool.

Mindfulness meditation is being taught in schools and workplaces, and as an adjunct to many different healthcare treatments, including cancer treatment. The evidence base for its effectiveness is extensive. Its effects include reducing cortisol and the effects of stress and, from the research of Elizabeth Blackwell, improving telomerase function and therefore cell longevity.

With growing acceptance of the situation I was facing, the life challenge that I was going through, and the ability to see my thoughts without judgement of them, it was explained to me that 'I am not my thoughts', that my thoughts were only what I was thinking, but who is the 'I' that is thinking those thoughts? That was the journey I was sent on, the discovery of that 'I', the understanding of myself and my values, and what would bring meaning and purpose in my life. This is the basis of the cornerstone of our spiritual health.

I will pick up the story of how I chose a valued direction, and what my action plan was in Chapter 10. Just to demonstrate how integrated our health truly is, the psychologist observed that I was overweight and that in order to regain psychological health, I also needed to build my physical health. In Latin, *mens sana in corpore sano*—'a healthy mind in a healthy body'. Although I was being treated for depression, the effect was that I was being taught tools for life, actually, as it turned out, tools for a life of flourishing.

Good work

Since psychological health depends on psychological safety and controlling thoughts of fear, this category also includes work. Work, particularly good work, is a key determinant of health. Not to detract from the value of voluntary work and parenting, work gives us financial security. Financial security is important as a way of escaping the harmful effects of poverty and the social determinants of health. At the positive end of the spectrum, work provides us with the means to fulfil our dreams and hopes, our life vision.

But not all work is good work. It was Dame Carol Black who pointed out to us that bad work is more harmful to health than no work at all. As an occupational physician, a doctor specializing in the health of work, the role of work in people's lives and the effect it has on their health is a central part of what I do. I work with employers to help them look after their workers. I work with unions to help them support the health of their members at work, and in discussions with employers.

What is good work? I believe it is provided by employers who respect their employees as people with lives outside work, with roles in their families and communities. Good employers keep workers safe from physical and psychological harm and reward them appropriately. Importantly, good employers don't tolerate bullying, harassment, and discrimination in the workplace. They implement policies to stamp them out. Given what we know from the importance of control in our lives, and the work of Sir Michael Marmot, good work provides a degree of autonomy, control, and flexibility over how people perform their work. Really good employers create a culture of health and provide programmes to support the health and wellbeing of their workers, resulting in greater engagement, reduced staff turnover, and higher productivity.

Poverty is known to be one of the key social determinants of health. But the converse is also true—financial security improves health. For all of us. The evidence is that money does bring happiness—just up to the level you feel financially secure. Beyond that, it loses its impact. Work supports financial security. In this section of my assessment, I therefore assess the degree to which you have financial health, and the strategies you can develop to gain control of your own financial security. This is important for both you and your family.

A lot of my work with clients involves helping them return to work after illness or injury. But it also includes encouraging people to better themselves at work. If dreams have not been fulfilled, what alternative actions could be taken?

Remember, the health gradient is a straight line: the better the quality of your job, the better the quality of your health. At the launch of the *Consensus Statement on the Health Benefits of Work*, Dame Carol Black made it abundantly clear that it is very much the role of doctors to support and encourage their patients to return to work and to gain the health benefits of work:

> Health professionals have a clear duty and responsibility to make this happen, and key roles to play. Those begin with promoting the necessary shifts in beliefs and understanding, and reversing the belief that we have to be totally fit and well to work or that recovery from illness or injury must be complete before return. Restoration of working life is closely aligned to clinical goals. It should be embedded in health professional judgements and in the drive to better the public health.[7]

Get this right and we improve the health of our communities and countries. And doctors have a fundamental role to play, which is not just to provide 'treatment'.

Work is a part of our lives, but it's an extremely important part, and is inextricably linked to our health, and indeed for many people, their fulfilment in life. Look at the PERMA model of wellbeing:

Positive emotions, including happiness
Engagement and flow
Relationships
Meaning
Achievement

It is very easy to see how work can both provide and add to all the components that Seligman sees as part of flourishing. Work can help you flourish in life!

I want to debunk the thinking behind the term 'work–life balance'. Work should be considered an integral part of our lives. Many people with disability seek support to help them return to work. For some people, their satisfaction in life, their quality of life, comes from activities other than paid work, such as parenting and volunteer work. But in Western society at least, work as an enabler of life and health should be fundamental. The balance to be struck is actually a balance between all components of our lives: work, family, leisure ('me time'), friends, exercise, and sleep. A tricky balance maybe, but the evidence is clear. Get the balance right and every single component of our lives can contribute positively to our health. My realization, after a decade of presenting on the health benefits of good work, is that there's a bigger picture: the health benefits of a good life. And it should be available to all of us.

We need healthcare and social care systems that empower people to take control of their lives and health to achieve the health benefits of a good life. Doctors can play key roles within those systems.

For me, my Positive Medicine Plan includes strategies for maintaining optimism and positivity, for prioritizing things that make me happy.

If you're feeling down, there's nothing worse than someone saying, 'Cheer up!' Yet it is also possible to look for a thought that's a bit better than you're feeling right now. Just keep it realistic.

I know what makes me happy. I know what will cheer me up if I'm feeling down. I've got a list of things I love, a lot of which are fulfilled by being in nature, and walking, especially by water. But also, being with family and friends, especially laughter over meals. And my hobbies: photography, reading, exercise, and yoga classes. Even chocolate, that's there too! (That's one I bring out in case of emotional emergency! It was given as a tip to me, and I regard it as invaluable.)

You know what some of the things on your list would be. Do yourself a favour; stop reading now and just scribble some notes. I quickly came up with 30 things I love. Having them written down makes it very easy to refer to them.

The great thing is that the list of things you love works however you may be feeling. Feeling good? Reach for your list of things you love and pick one or more. I guarantee you'll feel even better!

This is how having help in developing a plan impacted the psychological health of one of my clients:

Coming out of a complex collapse in my general wellbeing would not have been possible without professional help. I had become disconnected from myself, from others, and from the world in general, and I needed a framework, a plan to help me move back to feeling and being whole. As I worked with Dr David, I could feel a positive reintegration take place. Simple things, like writing down the 'why', 'how', and 'what' around practical steps I could take physically and emotionally, and then taking action and being accountable to my plan, rapidly brought a feeling of hope and wholeness back into my life. The sense of purpose that arose along with this hope and wholeness was largely what had been missing. I believe that building a plan that encompassed all aspects of my wellbeing was the major component in my recovery.

10

Emotional Health—Te Taha Whānau

Sir Mason Durie called this cornerstone of health after the family, whānau, because of the central nature of the family in Māori life. As I have mentioned, the word whānau denotes something bigger than the immediate family, and extends to communities.

Sir Mason stresses the family's important role as a support mechanism, and also as part of our sense of belonging. Maslow expands the concept, calling this tier of the pyramid the 'love needs', the need for affection, love, and sense of belonging. As well as the roots of health, he also believed 'the thwarting of these needs is the most commonly found core of maladjustment and more severe psychopathology'. Maslow saw that sexual needs, as well as being part of basic, physiological needs, also came into this tier, as part of the need for love and affection. In Seligman's theory of wellbeing, it is relationships that are key.

Certainly, for me, the breakdown of my marriage, the key relationship in my life, and the centre of the family, played a big role in the development of my emotional distress and subsequent mental ill health. But through the journey that followed, my realization of relationships could only strengthen. In the process, I rediscovered the sister who had been distanced from me (and I, her) by the circumstances of our childhood. I realized that my relationships with family and friends had to be a key part of my action plan and my habits for positive health going forward.

In my journey of self-discovery, I realized that Sir Mason was right, that the relationships with the wider family set the scene for our future health. The key relationship is between parents and children, and given everything that we have said about the effect of adverse childhood experiences, so many of these are dependent on the effects of parenting and the need to give unconditional love. As I look at my childhood and that of my sister, I realize that we were both adversely affected by aspects of it, particularly through religious influences.

But it's something that is common to many of my clients, and my friends. Even if we have not overtly experienced the terror that Maslow describes that many sufferers of adverse childhood experiences must have suffered, we have all been influenced adversely to one degree or another. Uncomfortable as it

Positive Medicine. David Beaumont, Oxford University Press. © Oxford University Press 2021.
DOI: 10.1093/oso/9780192845184.003.0011

feels, that means that we, as parents, are likely to have adversely influenced the health of our own children. But we do our best, with what we know, just as our parents did. In the words of the famous Philip Larkin poem:

> They fuck you up, your mum and dad.
> They may not mean to, but they do.
> They fill you with the faults they had
> And add some extra, just for you.[1]

I remember being introduced to the poem at school. We thought it was hilarious, because our teacher had to swear, but of course it's pretty dark too. Larkin apparently thought it a key concept for life, since he named it 'This be the verse'.

In the next verse, Larkin points out that our parents 'were fucked up in their turn'. Their parenting skills were learnt from their own experience. Our parents did the best they could with the level of knowledge they had. It is important for us to see how the influences of childhood have impacted how we see life and, indeed, how we parent our own children. We have choices: to repeat the patterns of past generations, or to learn and grow and do it differently. I was impacted for years by the realization that my father never told me that he loved me. It was only a few years ago, when my best mate told me that his father hadn't told him either, that I realized it was a generational thing—it just wasn't done, in the North of England, at that time. Rest assured I learnt from it and make a point of telling my own children, to this day.

The child is father to the man

There's a reason why the first 7 years of childhood are so important, and that is because that is when our brains are primed to learn exponentially. We soak up information like a sponge, not because we're processing it, but we are storing it. The prominent brain wave during these years is the very slow (0.5–4 cycles per second) theta wave. This is also the brain pattern that is achieved during hypnosis, which gives the clue as to where the information is going: into our subconscious minds. And just as in hypnosis, the information goes in unfiltered.

If a child is told they are bad, or stupid, then that is what they believe. And it stays with them, somewhere in the subconscious, and it affects their adult behaviours and attitudes. For me, it was the conflict between what I was being told about the purity of religion and people who shared the faith of my parents and my understanding that I was naughty. That conflict led to a deep-seated belief that I was bad, not good enough.

Our imprinted beliefs become either what triggers us into reacting (angrily, emotionally, fearfully), or, just as bad, become limiting beliefs that stop us from exploring and achieving our full potential: I'll never be able to do that, I'm not good enough. Knowing this gives us the roots to understand ourselves, and challenge and overcome our triggers and limiting beliefs. It also gives us a very, very good reason to try to be the best parents we can be. There's a lot of information on parenting out there. There's a lot to learn!

A key to addressing our triggers and limiting beliefs is through loving relationships. During my assessment with clients, I explore with them their loving relationships, and together we develop strategies. Loving relationships are another determinant of health, and again the converse is true, that loneliness is a killer. In illness, people often disengage from their family and friends, and the things they love to do. This compounds their illness, and needs to be reversed.

Be kind

Sadly, one of the key relationships damaged by childhood experiences is that with the self. If our key subconscious learning is that we're not good enough, not loveable, then inevitably it affects our love for ourselves. One of the key pieces of work we need to do is learn how to love ourselves. Not knowing how to love ourselves must affect our ability to love others or, more particularly, accept that someone else could love us, resulting in loss of self-esteem, self-belief, and self-confidence. At its worst, it results in self-loathing and self-harm. Clearly, at extremes, this requires professional support, and I would include psychological therapy in the action plan.

There is a technique that can be helpful, which is to set the intention that every day for 21 days you will preface every decision you make (even small, everyday ones) with the question, 'What would a person who loves themselves do?'

By taking the emotion out of the situation and making the decision a more conscious process, instead of a reactive, subconscious response, it increases the likelihood of habit formation and new habit development. Faced with criticism, what would a person who loves themselves do? Take on board anything constructive; if the criticism is not constructive, it says more about the other person than you. Faced with choices around food or alcohol, what would the person who loves themselves do? Make the healthy choice. Or, if not, be kind to themselves and not be self-critical.

Can you think of anything wrong with your partner? *Stop right there.* Don't go any further with that thought!

That's our tendency, isn't it? To look for fault. We've already established that not every love relationship is going to survive, and it takes bravery to end such a relationship. But sometimes we cloud our own opinion by looking for fault. Instead, here's an exercise: make a list of all the things you love about your partner, big things, little things, as many as you can. And share it with them. Tell them how much you appreciate them, and here are the reasons. Tell them you love them too, but by providing a list of evidence why you do, they are far more likely to be reassured.

Part of the positive medicine plan will include the steps the client is going to take to put effort into their relationship. Things like little spontaneous gifts or cards, planning a date night, the gift of some 'me time' for your partner. It's not hard, but it takes intention. This is also the part of the assessment where we consider sexual health.

As I have previously said, although this is an area that doctors find difficult to discuss, it is an area that's very important to patients. I find they are comfortable discussing it. My own comfort in discussing this fundamental part of people's life comes from very early in my general practice days. I must have been younger than 30 when an older couple came to me and said, 'Look, we do love each other, but our sex life has become very dull and boring, and often it's easier not to bother. What do you suggest?'

They clearly thought that the sexual health of patients was part of the role of a GP, and didn't expect me to feel uncomfortable. So I didn't. I just asked them what it had been like when it was good, what worked for each of them, and what didn't. I asked each of them, 'What would you like it to look like?'

That's all I did. I didn't tell them what to do, I just facilitated a conversation. They came up with the answers. Like so many areas in a patient's health, the patient knows better than anyone else in the world what the problem is and what success looks like. People just need enabling and empowering. The answers lie within.

My positive medicine plan includes a category on emotional health, which includes how I intend to relate to my family and friends, especially my children. How I can be the best dad, and also the best partner? It's geared to me being kind to myself and showing self-love, and also having my own needs met.

The process moves to relationships with the extended family and with work colleagues. As social beings, we need connections, and loving connections.

But, of course, at any of these levels of connection we might encounter strong relationships or those that challenge us and trigger negative responses.

There are many relationships and circumstances that can trigger us—that cause us to react defensively or even aggressively. Or passively and with resignation ('What's the point?'). If that happens, we could just accept that's who we are and how we react, which is probably therefore the conclusion that our friends have already reached. Or, we could challenge our own thinking. If we do find ourselves triggered then it usually means that our sense of identity has been challenged. Our ego feels threatened.

The US speaker and author Byron Katie believes that our root of suffering in this situation is believing our own thoughts to be true. She therefore designed a process to challenge our thinking, to reach a place of acceptance.

She calls her process 'The Work'. It's our own work to do; no one else's. Here are the stages:

- Notice or recall a situation that has angered or upset you.
- Write it down, as specifically as possible; time, place, person, who said what.
- Question it, objectively. Apply four questions:
  - Is it true?
  - Can you absolutely know it's true?
  - How do you react, what happens, when you believe that thought?
  - How would you be without that thought?
- What happens if you turn it around?
  - Could it be the opposite is true or truer than the original statement?[2]

Our triggers, our negative emotional reactions, are shaped by who we believe we are, and in turn influenced by the messaging that has reached our subconscious minds all the way from childhood; things said by our parents, teachers, television, and marketing. The younger we were, the less filtering our subconscious mind does, the more it believes it is true.

The underlying beliefs we develop as a result can be as bleak as 'I'm not worthy', 'I'm unlovable', or 'I'm not good enough'. They become the underpinning statements for our limiting beliefs; the subconscious barriers that hold us back from taking on life's challenges with confidence and self-belief. These become our stories, the stories we tell ourselves about who we are.

By doing The Work (repeatedly) we learn how to challenge our limiting beliefs. By turning the situation around and questioning which is more true, we begin to see it isn't just us, it's everyone who has limiting beliefs that don't serve them. 'John really upset me today' explored from the opposite becomes, 'I really upset John today'.

Why shouldn't that be just as true? Do you know what triggered John to react in the way he did towards you? Do you know what's happening in John's life today? Do you know that his mother has just been diagnosed with breast cancer? I'm sure if you did, you would have responded to the situation very differently, with acceptance and empathy. You would not have reacted defensively towards him.

If you find yourself triggered, find your anger or emotions rising, first: stop. Take a breath. Don't react, respond. Don't react with the first thought that came into your mind, but after the pause, respond with words that are more likely to calm the situation, or open up constructive dialogue. Recognize that if you are about to react emotionally, it is probably your own ego that is going into defensive mode, which will only cause you (and others) more suffering and pain.

Ego reactions don't serve us well. I believe there are three escalating levels of living and experiencing life and our relationship interactions that serve us. They add to our life experience and that of others:

- Accept and allow
- Experience and enjoy
- Excitement and passion

We cannot hope to be at that third, peak experience, tier all the time. But we can learn, I hope, at least to accept and allow the reactions of others, and accept them for what they are: their own triggers and ego defences.

Wholehearted living

Another expert in the understanding of how our lives shape our view of who we are is the social scientist and researcher Brené Brown. Her 2010 TED talk, 'The power of vulnerability', is one of the most accessed, with over 40 million views.[3] From her research into the feelings of shame and vulnerability that we develop through life experience, particularly from childhood, she came to realize that the acceptance and understanding of our own vulnerability actually becomes a strength. That once acknowledged, it no longer needs to limit and shape us. The point that acknowledgement enables us to reach she calls wholeheartedness:

Wholehearted living is about engaging in our lives from a place of worthiness. It means cultivating the courage, compassion, and connection to wake up in the morning and think, *No matter what gets done and how much is left undone, I am enough*. It's going to bed at night thinking, *Yes, I am imperfect and vulnerable and sometimes afraid, but that doesn't change the truth that I am also brave and worthy of love and belonging*.[4]

Developing emotional health involves exploring and building our relationships with the significant people in our lives. More importantly, it involves a process of self-exploration and acknowledgement of who we are: perfect in all our imperfections. By understanding our vulnerabilities and learning to approach life wholeheartedly, we can experience better-quality relationships and develop the courage to face life's challenges and embrace its opportunities. Within this also lies the roots of resilience—the bravery to face adversity and defeat, to pick ourselves up and start again. This is a characteristic shared by many people considered to be successful at life.

11

Spiritual Health—Te Taha Wairua

Sir Mason Durie referred to this cornerstone as 'spiritual health', and placed it as the most important of the four cornerstones for Māori, 'the most basic and essential requirement for health'.

I have come to understand why that is, but to explain why, I have to broaden the definition to encompass our search for meaning: why we are here, why we exist. Sir Mason makes clear that for Māori, te taha wairua may include religion, though not necessarily so. It also includes our relationship to our environment and the land, and to our ancestors (in common with many indigenous belief systems, for instance those of aboriginal peoples). It also includes the concept of *mana*.

I think it best to leave it to Sir Mason to define this word:

> Te taha wairua, the spiritual side of health, also accounts for a vital ingredient in the lives of some people, the presence of mana. Mana has been variously translated as self-esteem, personal prestige, charisma, but unlike those states it does not derive from a person's strengths or individual pursuit. Instead, it is a state conferred by the gods, a state of spiritual authority and power, denoting a high level of spiritual core without an egocentric core. To possess mana is to know health.

This resonates with the corresponding tier of Maslow's hierarchy, the esteem needs. Maslow felt that, before we could start to address esteem needs fully, we needed the other tiers of the pyramid to be met. We all have a need for a stable base of self-esteem, self-respect, and feelings of esteem for others. He saw us as needing acknowledgement of our capacities, achievements, and adequacy (we need to be seen to be good enough, by ourselves as well as others), and with this recognition comes a sense of confidence to face the world, including facing life's challenges, in order to gain independence and freedom, a sense 'of being useful in the world'.

This is where I see Martin Seligman's two categories of meaning and accomplishment: a feeling that what we are doing is meaningful and that we are

Positive Medicine. David Beaumont, Oxford University Press. © Oxford University Press 2021.
DOI: 10.1093/oso/9780192845184.003.0012

accomplishing something worthwhile. I think too the engagement he sees us finding when we are truly engrossed in what we love to do arises because we find it fulfilling, and find ourselves in a state of flow.

The *Oxford Textbook of Spirituality in Healthcare* describes spirituality as 'a subjective experience that exists both within and outside traditional religious systems. It relates to the way in which people understand and live their lives in view of their sense of ultimate meaning and value. Spirituality in this sense includes the need to find satisfactory answers to ultimate questions about the meaning of life, illness, and death. It can be seen as comprising elements of meaning, purpose, value, hope, relationships, love, and for some people, a connection to a higher power or something greater than self.'[1]

We know that doctors find it difficult to discuss spirituality, probably because they confuse it with religion (and possibly patients do too), although patients do want to be able to discuss purpose and meaning in life. For that reason, I also term this cornerstone 'existential health'. Existentialism is concerned with the uniqueness of the human experience, living lives of meaning and purpose, with a sense of freedom to choose and live with passion, sincerity, and authenticity. Although that is how I've come to regard spirituality, in its broadest sense, I hope that existential health is something we can agree we all need to some degree, even if we have defined it fully for ourselves.

My journey of self-discovery came out of adversity, and particularly from my experience of depression. For me, it consolidated the concept that is the premise of this book, that medical practice is not just about treatment and recovery, it is about healing. Healing must involve all four cornerstones of our health, which are inextricably linked. Both healing and health are words which come from the Old English word 'haelan' which means to make whole. To integrate our four cornerstones and become whole is how we achieve healing.

The journey was prompted by my psychologist, who helped me understand that I am not my thoughts. So, who is the 'I' who is thinking? We know when we are thinking, we can observe ourselves thinking. It's a challenging philosophical concept, but who knows we are thinking? Who is observing our thoughts? That is the inner self, the true self.

It has been an amazing journey, and the route continues to unfold before me. It also encompasses the wisdom of the ages. The Ancient Greek aphorism, 'Know thyself', was inscribed in the Temple of Apollo at Delphi, and later asserted by the classical Greek philosopher, Socrates.

The tasks I worked through in therapy, through the modality known as ACT (acceptance and commitment therapy), were:

Accept the situation and be present in the moment.
Choose a valued direction: I had to define my values and find my purpose.
Take action.

Having developed the practice of mindfulness meditation, accepted my situation and my life challenges, the next step was to define my values. I went to a stationery shop and bought paper and coloured pens, which I spread out on the table, ready for the exercise. I sat down and wrote:

Be true to myself.
Be there for my family and friends.
Make a difference.

That was it. The whole exercise took me 30 seconds.

Having identified my values, my next job was to define my purpose and start to take action. By then, my concepts for a more whole-person model of medical practice were starting to coalesce, even if there was still work to be done refining them. But I knew it was my purpose: to change the model of medical practice. That was my audacious goal.

By that time, I was doing conference presentations on the health benefits of good work and was describing health as being more than the absence of disease. I knew that an action step I needed was to undertake a course in public speaking, so I joined Toastmasters. Being put on the spot and critiqued for something that people inherently find uncomfortable and scary is really helpful for gaining confidence. One evening we had the ultimate on-the-spot and, potentially, 'die-on-the-stage' experience. We had to stand up in front of the group, one by one, and deliver a presentation on the spot. And we didn't know the topic until we stood up.

My turn came. The Chair said, 'OK David, talk for 5 minutes on the topic of … religion.'

The unprepared presentation has to be entertaining and informative, so there isn't time to filter anything you say. To add a note of humour (extra points from the group!) I started by explaining, tongue in cheek, that I was a 'devout atheist' and had been since childhood, ever since being raised in a very strict Christian denomination, one that believed in the Bible completely literally, word for word. I explained how this did not fit with my early interest in science and biology, and how my rejection of religion at an early age was a disappointment to my mother. It was easy to fill 5 minutes with unfiltered thoughts and feelings, and I was scored highly.

On the way home, I suddenly started laughing, at the realization of what I had said. I had totally rejected the literal description of the events of the Bible, and could not fathom the concept of an old man with a long grey beard called God who sat on a cloud and dished out blessings or punishment (seriously, exactly the image I had from my 7-year-old self, I can see the picture now). For that reason, I had spent my whole life staunchly believing in … nothing! How ridiculous it felt at that moment. But humorous too, and therefore exciting.

The search for the meaning of my existence could begin in earnest.

Having told you that the clients I see are happy to talk about their own belief systems with me, there was one who wasn't.

She said, 'I'm sorry, that makes me feel really uncomfortable. It's not something I want to talk about.'

She explained that she had been brought up in a very religious family and had rejected their belief system. I immediately empathized, and said I had too, and that had shaped my own response to considering issues of matters bigger than us.

The next session we had, she explained further. Deep down she knew that she did have a belief system, but her discomfort, she realized, was precisely because it conflicted with the family viewpoint. But she had realized that actually it was probably the most important thing she needed to do, to reconcile those positions and start her journey of self-discovery.

It was very exciting to be part of those reflections with her, as my client developed the strategy of whom she was going to talk to, what she was going to read, and what she was going to ask of herself in meditation.

Getting to know Matey

My own journey of self-discovery took a fascinating twist while I was in recovery from depression. It was before my hip replacement. I was still in pain from my hip osteoarthritis, and I wasn't sleeping well, accompanied by a common symptom of depression, early morning waking. I was on holiday in the UK, in the northern summer, and at 4 am the sun was shining brightly. What else could I do but go for a walk?

As I walked along the banks of the River Trent that morning, the birds were singing, the wildflower meadows were blooming in abundance, and the odd butterfly was already warming its wings. I suddenly realized how strongly this all resonated with me, how it reminded me of my childhood. There was woodland at the bottom of our garden, with a stream flowing through the valley. As a young child I would spend hours down there, playing by myself. I loved nature, and I knew the name of every bird, every wildflower, every butterfly. (I had pestered my parents to get me nature books to identify them.) I had forgotten how important being in nature was to me. It seemed like another life (it was a long time ago!), but the more I reflected, the more I realized it wasn't, it was me. In fact, it was *real me*. I could visualize lying on the grassy bank on a balmy summer's day, just watching the clouds scud by. Although I had already begun to be indoctrinated by (and to reject) religion, this little boy represented to me the purest form of me.

Over the weeks that went by, I realized that I could recall more experiences as a 7-year-old than I had thought. And they were *my* experiences. I remembered being in Miss Haigh's class, as a 7-year-old, and writing about a TV programme I had watched over the weekend. It was a black-and-white, BBC Open University programme on science and nature. I was hooked. I wrote about cells and 'monocules'. Even now I can see Miss Haigh's red line and her correction to 'molecules' in the margin, and the conversation she had with my parents about encouraging me. They subsequently bought me a basic microscope, the first of three over the next few years. I can still vividly see the scene from the black-and-white TV programme. Two lecturers were demonstrating the 'monocule' using wooden beads and dowelling. Looking back, I realized that this was the double-helix shape of the DNA molecule.

I may have known by the age of 11 that I was going to be a doctor, but the seeds were already sown at the age of 7.

I came to know that little boy as Matey, which was the name my dad called me when he came home from work. 'Hi Matey, how was your day?'

I knew that Matey didn't fit in with the people around him, and that he often felt very alone in that conflict between science and religion; but I used to tell him it was OK, that he would become a doctor, that his dreams would be fulfilled.

Only recently I came to discover that this technique is actually used as a form of therapy, known as 'inner child work', which originated from the concepts of Swiss psychiatrist and psychoanalyst Carl Jung. For me, it was not only part of my journey of self-discovery, but also part of my healing from depression. Since that time, I have been able to trace the threads of that little boy in my persona through the many different phases of my life. He is me, an integral part of me, and I can connect with that part of me in meditation. That still small voice that is my true self, the real me. I have not shared my developing belief system with you, the reader, because everyone's journey will take them to different interpretations of meaning and purpose for them, but to be true to myself I felt I needed to share the story of Matey. The realization that there is an inner self who reflects my essence, my true self, and is a part of me I can connect with at any time in meditation has been a revelation to me.

I am privileged in my assessments to have clients to share their life stories with me. One, named Glyn, has had to change career after an injury. He's decided to fulfil his dream of being a farmer. Only today, Glyn was reflecting on one of the actions he is progressing from his Life and Health Integration Plan. As part of his recovery from a brain injury, he decided that he needed to read more. He picked a book from his childhood, *The Children of the New Forest*, by Frederick Maryat. The book was worn and musty, but even the smell was evocative of his childhood. The inside front cover was inscribed by his Sunday school teacher. He had won it as a prize. He vividly recalled asking his father what certain words meant.

He is reading it slowly and deliberately, savouring every chapter, as the last thing he does each evening. He told me that recently, as he put the book down quietly, he recalled an event in his young, 8-year-old life. It was April 1968. His father was working on the Lyttelton to Wellington ferry, the *Wahine*. It left Lyttelton Harbour in bad weather, which by the time they arrived at Wellington had become one of the worst storms in New Zealand's history. The ship hit a reef at the harbour entrance and foundered, with the eventual loss of 53 lives. Because of the storm, lines of communication were lost. The family didn't know if their father was among the lost.

Several days later there was a knock at the door. Glyn vividly recalled a man in uniform handing his mother a telegram. She went into the room to read it. He remembered her tears as she read the two words it contained: 'AM SAFE.'

His father had got into a lifeboat, which immediately overturned in the waves. The tugboat *Tapuhi* tried to pick up survivors. His father's colleague was sucked into the boat's propeller and perished. The other boat which arrived on the scene, a pilot boat, picked up Glyn's father and other passengers.

As my client told me the story, it was clear he had found his inner child. The experience was totally real to him; as though he was back there experiencing the lived experience all over again. He knew he was that child. That child has also been there, within him. His true self. He still has that telegram.

Best me

I continue my journey of self-discovery on a daily basis. I continue to gain new insights, and am loving the journey of my life. I have definitely experienced dis-ease in my life, and disease, and illness and chronic pain.

Right now, I feel healthier than I have for a long, long time. I am at the ease end of the spectrum, I'm loving life. I can't easily think back to a time when I had no pain, but right here, right now, I have no pain. I have my own Life and Health Integration Plan and I try to follow the positive health habits that it con-tains. The health benefits of being in nature have now been well documented, as contained in the *Oxford Textbook of Nature and Public Health*,[2] and I walk in nature as often as I can. I also try to do mindfulness meditation on a daily basis. I have defined for me what my goals are for my ideal physical health, psychological health, emotional health, and spiritual health. I have developed a number of mantras I use in meditation, to help instil the feeling of integra-tion that combining all four cornerstones suggests. I don't mind sharing one of them with you (as long as you realize that it's aspirational!):

> I am Best Me:
> Best Body
> Best Mind
> Best Heart
> Best Soul
> Best Me.

As we have seen, Maslow's theory of human motivation held that we are all driven to be the best we can be, to self-actualize, that is the ultimate motiva-tion. But to fulfil that, we have to see ourselves as humans living lives in which our environment, particularly the effects of childhood, will impact our ability to fulfil our needs. Maslow defined a hierarchy of those needs, within which meeting each tier was the basis for addressing higher needs. To have those needs thwarted was to risk developing psychopathy—mental ill health.[3]

It turns out that Maslow was right, but he didn't go far enough. It also causes physical pathology, illness, and disease. And we now have started to under-stand the epigenetic and neuroimmunological mechanisms by which these develop.

But Maslow was less concerned about the pathology and far more concerned about how this understanding could be used to the good, to positive effect. After all, he obtained his understanding from people who were successful, who were flourishing in life. He presented a list of 13 underlying premises that formed the basis of his theory. The first he called 'The integrated whole-ness ... of the foundation stones of motivation theory'.[4]

I have deliberately aligned Maslow's four lower tiers with the four corner-stones of the Māori model of health. They align, are concordant, they support each other, and for many overlapping reasons. No matter which way I look at it, and despite Martin Seligman insisting to me that to flourish is not the same as to self-actualize, I think it's the closest modern equivalent. It is certainly more easily understood by the generations coming through who may not necessarily feel that self-actualization is a term they understand, has anything to do with them, or may be achievable for them.

On the other hand, to say to someone of the modern generations (that is, everyone reading this book, by the way) that to integrate all these four do-mains of your life, the four cornerstones of your health, will enable you to flourish ... now surely that's something worth having? And to have a plan to achieve it, to achieve 'integrated wholeness' that leads to healing.

So, here's the question. If I have been my own (initially unwitting) experi-mental subject, has it worked for me?

Flourishing

I must admit to a certain reticence in writing this, but throughout this book I have shared with you my very personal lows, and therefore it would be incom-plete for me not to share the highs.

Looking at the four cornerstones of my health: my physical health has not been better for decades. Absolutely, modern medicine has played a major role in that, but my measures of homeostasis, my blood pressure, blood chemistry, and basic functioning are good. My psychological health? Well, any semblance of depression is long gone. I'm in a state of ease, and yes, I'm very happy with my life. Emotional health: I'm in a wonderful love relationship, and my rela-tionship with my children is fantastic. I'm so proud of them and they know it. I have wonderful friends (even if some of them are distant, in the UK).

Could I do better? Yes, absolutely. We're not aiming for perfect, we're aiming for continuous improvement, to continue to be better. I could be there more for my sister in the UK, who could do with some support right now.

Spiritual or existential health? I have never been more clear about who I am, why I'm here, and where I'm going. For me, the exploration of my journey of self-discovery has been astounding, and continues to be. While

I continue to explore inwards, I devour books by others who are exploring, and books on wellbeing and the new sciences. There are so many new and exciting developments in how we understand how we function as integrated whole people. I watch videos and TED talks by very, very clever people who are pushing our thinking further and further.

Why are we here (the ultimate existential question)? Everyone will reach a different conclusion, but for me, I would say it is to experience life joyfully, and to help others to experience life joyfully.

Self-actualization I see as a state you go in and out of. What do you do when you've become the best you can be? You realize you can get even better.

So, of the characteristics that Maslow identified, how do I fare? Join me in going through the list of Maslow's characteristics and experiences of people who do self-actualize, who do become the best they can be. It must always be an evolution, but I do believe that many people do get glimpses of what self-actualization looks and feels like. That realization surely is a driver to want to experience more. That's what Maslow believed—that this is the ultimate motivator.

Critical thinking—an astute perception of reality and ability to reason.

I think that's what I've been trying to do for the last 20 years of working through the conundrum I saw of what is not working about modern medicine.

Acceptance of imperfection—accepting and non-judging of themselves and others.

My psychologist taught me a lot about acceptance, since it is the underlying premise of ACT. We are our own worst critics; we judge ourselves the harshest. In fact, when we judge other people's behaviour, it often says more about us than it does about them! So yes, I have become much more accepting of myself and others through this journey.

Spontaneous—willing to take risks and experience life to the full.

Hell yes, bring it on!

Higher purpose—they see a problem and feel driven to resolve it, more to the benefit of other people than themselves, 'a task they must do'.

Aha. This is it. This book brings together the concepts that constitute my higher purpose. My higher purpose is to build a new model of medical practice. Maslow said, 'What a man can be, he must be.' That's how I feel right now.

Comfortable with being alone—a strong sense of autonomy and a calmness and confidence in their own abilities. Self-directed.

After my marital separation I went through a phase of feeling very alone, very lonely. My realization was through my work getting to re-know my inner child, Matey. He spent hours alone, down by the stream. He loved his own company and his own thoughts. Now, so do I. And yes, I feel in control of my own destiny and clear about what I need to do.

Fresh appreciation—they seem to be able to always appreciate and express gratitude for their life experiences.

I'm loving the experience of life. My development of the habits of positive health has taught me the need to express gratitude. I try to incorporate it into my daily meditation practice. It's not hard at all to say thank you for that wonderful dinner with friends, and the fun and laughter we had; although it's not always easy to remember to reflect and deliberately express gratitude at the end of the day. It's a lot harder to express gratitude for things that go wrong. But that's where true peace comes from, when you can realize what the learning and the benefit was. I've had quite a few tough times over the last few years, but every one of them has made me stronger and more thankful (eventually!). This one is always a work in progress!

Peak experiences—there is a common description of the moments of high excitement, harmony, and deep meaning, even if only momentary.

For me, it is always about nature. Because these experiences are inherently so personal, you may not get this. Sometimes, when I'm out for a walk by the lake and I realize that there, just next to me at the water's edge in the reeds, is a mother duck with six new ducklings. They are playing together and oblivious of me, even though I'm only a few feet away. I get a completely overwhelming feeling of emotion. A feeling that right here, right now, this moment is perfect. That everything is well with the world. That it's all worthwhile. It gives me waves of goose bumps. (As you will have gathered, for me, that moment, that appreciation represents something deeply meaningful, and therefore, spiritual.)

For you, a peak experience might be a religious experience, or maybe the surge of emotion and adrenaline at a sporting event. Some people have peak experiences listening to a musical concert. For others, it is being in the flow as they paint or write or make something creative.

Connectedness—they have a strong sense of compassion and caring for others and a genuine desire to help others.

This is a common characteristic of doctors and other healthcare professionals, by virtue of their calling to do that work. For me, the highest experience I have felt of this was in the closing comments of Congress 2019, when I reminded the audience of the sub-theme, 'Ko Tātou, Tātou. We Are One', and the final words: 'In every healthcare interaction there is a person with their own life story, treating a person with their own life story.'

In that moment, with tears in my eyes, I knew we were all connected; all share the same suffering, the same joy, the same desire to make the experience better for ourselves and others.

Humility and respect—treating all people as equal; friendly and open with all.

I absolutely believe we're all equal. I value the contribution that other people make to my life—not just friends, but especially people providing a service to me. I have fantastic conversations with taxi drivers and restaurant waiting staff. I find taxi drivers in particular add to my life, and I hope I add to theirs. I always sit in the front passenger seat. For a captive few minutes, they often seem to love to share snippets from their life experience: where in the world they have come from, what they used to do, and how their family are doing. In those moments we touch each other's lives.

Sense of humour—able to laugh at themselves. Non-judgemental in their humour towards others.

Laughter among friends is one of the most satisfying of our experiences, isn't it? I'm sure I'm less sensitive to being the butt of a joke than I used to be. I've also got used to my children no longer being able to laugh at my dad jokes. On the other hand, I can always get 5-year-olds to howl with laughter at some of the old jokes, even if my children can only groan.

Life has thrown its curve balls at me, as it does for us all. I absolutely believe I have grown from the experience of having to pick myself up and dust myself down and just get on with it. I am now consciously on a journey to embrace the concept of growth and personal improvement. Glimpses of self-actualization does mean that I want to experience more. And in the process, I do believe I have developed the skills to adapt and self-manage in the face of life's challenges. The new definition of health—positive health. I hope you can see how you might be able to seize control of your life to achieve the same.

There's a further phase to positive medicine that I haven't mentioned yet, and that's the 5-year life vision. Once a client is working through their Life and Health Integration Plan and gaining confidence in their ability to take control of their life and health, I start the process of getting them to think what they want their life to look like in 5 years' time. What are the opportunities? (One client said, 'Oh my goodness, that's when the children leave home. I must plan for that, make the most of the opportunity and not get empty nest syndrome!')

Ask yourself: what do I need to do to achieve those opportunities? What do I want in my life and what do I *not* want? Am I settling for good enough, when my life could be so much better?

Working together, I help my clients develop their life vision. Suddenly, this creates an air of excitement, of possibility, an added layer of motivation.

I've known the culmination of my vision for a number of years now. It's looking more achievable, taking shape more feasibly as I journey. Within the next 5 years, I want to develop a health and healing centre. A place where people come to join with others in a dedicated venue to help them achieve integration, wholeness, and healing. Working in partnership with doctors and coaches.

In his book *The Road Less Travelled*, the US psychiatrist Dr M. Scott Peck points out that there are many different paths our lives can take. He sees the majority of people settling for *good enough* (or sadly, in some cases, bad enough). The road less travelled is often not the straightforward one. It takes courage to make tough decisions. But, he says, the rewards are there for the taking.[5]

There is an air of inevitability about middle age, a tendency to feel that it's downhill from here. Never mind, there's always retirement to look forward to. I don't know about your parents, but my parents were old at 50. That's what was expected; there was an expectation of how you looked, acted, dressed, behaved, and spoke, that was in keeping with being 50.

What we know now is that ageing is a choice, that life is a choice. There's no right or wrong, and no judgement, but you do need to be made aware of your choices. What we do now know is that there is a whole new science of ageing, and our understanding of ageing is now likely to expand exponentially.

We tell ourselves stories, of who we are, of what our life is, of what will happen in our lives. Pessimists tell one story; optimists another. The optimists live longer, happier, and healthier lives. Our stories are shaped significantly by our childhood, then by our life experiences on the way, but a big part of our story is actually what other people have told us is our story, or what they think our story should be. Our parents, teachers, bosses, the media, and advertising all shape our thinking. They aim to, it's deliberate! This is the root cause of our limiting beliefs, this very process that we're all put through. Every day of our lives. But we can still apply critical thinking to filter what is being said to us. We can question and challenge—just because someone says something about us, is it true? It doesn't have to be. It probably isn't.

Every good story has a victim, a villain, and a hero. If you look at the stories that become Hollywood blockbusters, the main character starts out a victim of circumstances. Life is tough and unfair, and they encounter adversity. While there's usually a villain in the piece who torments our hero, sometimes there's a twist in the story and they become the villain themselves, do something out of character. But then they overcome their self-doubt, realize the path they need to take, become the hero, and live happily ever after.

We like those stories. There are aspects we can relate to, because we're all on a journey of life. The stories we tell ourselves influence what that life looks like, and influence how we make life decisions, whether we decide to remain the victim or the villain, or whether we choose to take control and become the hero.

My partner's purpose is to help people change their stories; to realize that they can re-evaluate the plot line that they have been following so far; that they can learn skills, tactics, and strategies to see what's happened so far in a different light; and realize that the ending they had seen isn't set in stone, and that they can write the next chapter of their lives.

Here's the challenge for you. If you put aside your limiting beliefs, discount practicality, and don't worry about resources, what could your story ending look like? Dare to dream. Consider 'What if . . .?' Let your imagination run wild.

Be realistic, you're still you. If you're 55 and your dream was to play for the All Blacks, then that ship sailed long ago. But don't *artificially* limit yourself. There are infinite possibilities out there as to how your life might turn out. The potential for your life, therefore, is infinite. It's all about choice, so right now you can start making choices that take you towards that dream ending.

Here's the amazing news—all the evidence in this book points towards one conclusion: that to take control of your life, to believe that you control your destiny, to make choices that take you towards your dream, will dramatically increase your chances of living a longer, healthier, and happier life.

Maybe I should leave the closing words to my client Glyn:

I just keep reading through my plan. I just love reading it. It uplifts me. I really feel I know where I'm going now. I'm putting my heart and soul into getting my life back on track.

Epilogue

A Response to Ivan Illich

In the 1970s, Ivan Illich warned doctors that, by medicalizing the suffering of life which we all experience, doctors were robbing people of the ability to take control of their own lives. He set out his thesis in a book called *Medical Nemesis*.[1] By using medication to give people false hope that the effects of pain, of suffering, and of ageing and death could be mitigated, doctors, he predicted, would become the agents of their own demise. He even provided the evidence that it was happening.

Illich could not have been more provocative. He said that the greatest threat to people's health is doctors. He called it *iatrogenesis*[2]; it begins with the healer.

More than 40 years later, there is still dispute about how much death and disability doctors cause. Some say that to call it the third greatest cause of death after heart disease and cancer is an exaggeration. Others say that's an underestimate, and that it is actually the number one cause of death in the Western world.

Twenty years after writing *Medical Nemesis*, Ivan Illich reflected that the book had prompted 'shock and anger' when it was published in the 1970s. He reconsidered his views in the 1990s, and decided that, if anything, the assertions he had made were more true. But there was a specific part that he got wrong, he decided. In proposing that the solution was the empowerment of people to take control of their own lives and health, he had completely underestimated the power of the system. In 1994, in the preface to a new edition of the book, he wrote, 'In *Limits to Medicine—Medical Nemesis*, I argued that the fundamental pathogen today is the pursuit of health as this has come to be culturally defined in late-industrial society. I did not understand that in the age of systems management, this pathogenic pursuit of health would become universally imposed.'[3]

The shock and anger of doctors was completely understandable. To them, what Illich was accusing them of was so blatantly wrong, because it flew in the face of everything they had been taught in the heyday of medical science. They

Positive Medicine. David Beaumont, Oxford University Press. © Oxford University Press 2021.
DOI: 10.1093/oso/9780192845184.003.0013

took a strong defensive position and disagreed with him. They raged against Illich and the other voices in the 1970s who were sounding the alarm bell about the direction in which medicine was heading.

By completely disregarding Illich and others, the medical establishment fought off the challenge. The dogma of the medical model prevailed. But they didn't know the man; didn't know what drove him. All they saw was the threat he posed to their view of medicine. They didn't heed the warning of impending medical nemesis.

For that is what it was, a warning. It was a call to action, a wake-up call for people to see what was really happening. That's the way Illich worked. Modern medicine was far from his only challenge; he took the same approach with education, work, energy use, transportation, and economic development. In his critique of the modern education system, *Deschooling Society*, he challenged educationalists to reconsider the formulaic approach to systematizing education, and its contribution to the institutionalization of society.[4] He proposed a far more holistic and individual approach to learning which would become life-long. Thank goodness that at least the teachers and educationists listened to him.

Or did they? One of the most watched TED talks of all time, Sir Ken Robinson's 2006 talk 'Do schools kill creativity?' echoes many of Illich's themes in relation to the flaws of modern education. Again, decades after Illich sounded the warning.[5]

I personally recognize Illich as a disruptor. I recognize him, because I have to own that I am a disruptor too. Here's a dictionary definition of disruptor: 'Someone or something that interrupts an event, activity, or process by causing a disturbance or problem.' But there's a level of meaning beyond that. What the establishment didn't realize was that Illich was *deliberately* disrupting to prompt a response that would lead to a better outcome. In modern terminology, he was a *positive disruptor*: 'Someone who challenges current organizational habits and works to find positive alternatives; uprooting and changing how we think, behave, do business, learn and go about our day-to-day.'[6]

Illich's solution was for people to rise up and seize control of their own lives and health, collectively. People should change the system, should rise up against the expropriation of their health, and the removal of their ability to manage their own health by their subjugation to doctors. What he came to realize was that the power of the medical and pharmaceutical system negated any possibility of that being the solution. The patient–doctor relationship in the 1970s was inherently power-based, and the power imbalance between doctor and patient was based on knowledge. Under that paternalistic approach, doctors said, essentially, 'I know your health better than you do.'

In the 1970s, Dr Marshall Marinker wrote a response to *Medical Nemesis*. Marinker was already an influential GP when I did my GP training in the mid 1980s. By the time of his death in 2019, he was described as 'one of the notable GPs of the past half century in the UK'.[7] Of *Medical Nemesis* he wrote, 'I shall need to acknowledge and celebrate much of the analysis of the medical profession which Ivan Illich makes, and yet to challenge what seem to me to be unsatisfactory conclusions.'[8]

Marinker was a positive disruptor too. He also saw the flaws in the training of doctors, stating, 'There is a hidden curriculum in medical education that is based not on the medical school's declared intentions, but on the clinical behaviour of its teachers.'[9]

But I believe that he missed the point of Illich's conclusions, which he saw as idealistic and utopian. 'I suggest a society without unhealth would not be a utopia but a particular type of hell.' Contradicting his own assessment, he still concluded powerfully:

Medical Nemesis, whatever its author intends, must become part of the text for a reform of the medical curriculum. That some contemporary students, confronted with the model of medical care which their teachers present, can say, 'I am no longer sure that I want to be a doctor. I don't want to be like you' provides some evidence that the reform may be already upon us.[10]

Marinker's prediction of imminent reform was wrong, but only in timing. It took decades before that reform occurred. The modern medical curriculum, certainly here in New Zealand, is very different from the one that I and my contemporaries were taught. The doctor of the future will be far more like the doctor that Illich saw, and the person–doctor partnership will redress the power imbalance he warned against.

My overwhelming conclusion is that, in their fear of threat of change, doctors didn't hear Illich. If anyone could have heard, it was Marshall Marinker, but even he missed the point. In accusing Illich of painting a utopian future, he had not registered the conclusion to the summary of *Medical Nemesis* which Illich wrote for *The Lancet*, in which he explicitly stated:

The recovery of a health attitude towards sickness is neither Luddite nor Romantic nor Utopian: it is a guiding ideal which can never be fully achieved, which can be achieved with modern devices as never before in history, and which must orient politics to avoid encroaching Nemesis.[11]

Illich wanted doctors to avoid their nemesis. He saw there was a solution that was best for society, but he was also protective of the scarce (and expensive) resource that are doctors. He brought in the concepts of equity, empowerment, and responsibility. In truth, the model he presented meets all the requirements for being disruptive innovation: both better and cheaper than the established way. Illich wrote:

> The level of public health corresponds to the degree to which the means and responsibility for coping with illness are distributed among the total population. This ability to cope can be enhanced but never replaced by medical intervention or the hygienic characteristics of the environment. That society which can reduce professional intervention to the minimum will provide the best conditions for health. The greater the potential for autonomous adaptation to self, to others, and to the environment, the less management of adaptation will be needed or tolerated.[12]

Illich was overtly calling for health systems to move towards health enhancement, to achieve greater population health as well as individual control over life and health. He even saw health as the ability to adapt to changing circumstances: the new definition of positive health which was only realized by doctors nearly four decades later.

Recently, I was presenting to a group of doctors about the concepts in this book and the science behind the connection between medicine, health, and wellbeing. When they realized the book was still being written, they asked that I include two additional points. First, they pointed out that there is much being said about the harm (iatrogenesis) caused by doctors, and much 'doctor-bashing'. They felt badly done by. They pointed out that doctors are only fulfilling the role set for them by society, and in delivering medical care to patients they are providing the service that is expected. In other words, patients are complicit in the wrongs of the current model. Their second point was that the practice that doctors provide is decided by the healthcare system. The system is designed around a particular model of practice, so it is extremely hard to do anything but provide that model of care. To my mind, there is an even stronger third point: that senior doctors in particular are delivering only what they were trained to deliver. Like our parents in raising us, they are doing their best with their current level of knowledge.

I explained to them that there are a number of underlying premises for my book, as follows:

- Life course theory demonstrates that not only does our health affect our life, but life affects our health.
- There is new scientific evidence that identifies the role that environment and our choices have on our health (and sickness), including epigenetics and positive psychology.
- If we can develop the belief that we can take control of own lives and destiny, self-efficacy, we can improve our health and live longer and happier lives.
- The way that doctors have been trained during the era of advances in medical science has limited the evolution of the practice of medicine.

Our medical students are now being taught new science and new models of practice with compassion, but if we don't create the environment in which they can work to new models, it will be a long time before the new models are incorporated into practice. The dogma of the medical model from senior doctors is entrenched. It withstands logical and evidential challenge.

The field of psychology is changing, with two models of practice running in parallel. Traditional psychology deals with mental ill health, while positive psychology takes people from a state of coping to one in which they can flourish.

The definition of health has evolved. A new definition is that health is the ability to adapt and self-manage in the face of life's challenges. The proposal is for the new definition to be known as positive health. Life's challenges affect us all, at all stages of our life. Our body responds to challenge with defence systems developed through millennia of human evolution. The body's defence systems are mediated through the nervous and immune systems, under the central control of primitive parts of the brain which are not under conscious control, but influenced by our higher centres. Under states of unrelenting threats or challenges, particularly when primed by adverse childhood experiences, our nervous system and immune systems are unable to return to a normal state of balance, or ease in the system (homeostasis). Instead, a low-grade inflammatory state of allostasis, or dis-ease develops. This has the propensity to turn into illness or disease. Increasingly, this is being seen as the root of the majority of sickness in our society.

A model of medical practice is proposed which does not substitute for the medical model, but rather goes beyond it. It is meta medicine. It is not alternative or complementary, but mainstream. It is the third way. It is a model based on traditional Māori cultural views of health being an integrated whole: physical, psychological, whānau (family) or emotional health, and spiritual health. In order to present a concept that is universally acceptable, in the model I propose, 'spiritual' is added to 'existential' health. Maslow's hierarchy of needs, and theory of motivation, identifies that we are all driven by a desire to become the best we can be, which also coincides with those parts of life that bring purpose and meaning. The ultimate goal of humans is described by Maslow as self-actualization: becoming the person we were meant to be. In positive psychology, the ultimate state of being is known as flourishing. If the terms 'self-actualization' and 'flourishing' are not precisely synonymous, they are at the very least complementary.

Because the model relies on accurate diagnosis and prognosis, with the application of the medical model as a first stage, this model of practice is a truly medical model because doctors are uniquely qualified to practise it, even though it goes beyond their current training. Reaching a diagnosis will rely on the ability to distinguish conditions for which a specific pathological diagnosis can be reached from those for which investigations are negative and have been termed 'medically unexplained symptoms'. The new term of bodily distress disorder has now given these conditions a specific diagnostic label. It provides a mechanistic explanation for the symptom complexes being due to disorders of physiological function in the interaction between brain, nervous system, and immune system, at the dis-ease end of the spectrum. This allows for positive diagnosis, rather than diagnosis by exclusion after a myriad of tests have been conducted. It prevents people from feeling they are being labelled as having something that's 'all in your head'. The potential association between these conditions and the pre-existence of adverse childhood experiences and other traumatic circumstances is now being established.

To distinguish this new model of practice from traditional medicine, and to align it with the new definition of positive health and the science of positive psychology, I propose that it be called 'positive medicine'. The application of the model to form an individualized health plan (Life and Health Integration Plan) involves the incorporation of the habits of positive health into all aspects of the life of the individual, together with specification of what brings meaning and purpose (and therefore motivation) uniquely for that person.

What does this mean for patients?

The first part of the answer to this question is to go back to what patients want. Patients tell us they want to be upskilled to understand their own health; to be treated like an individual, not a collection of symptoms; and to be empowered to manage their own health. They want holistic care that recognizes the importance of the many facets of their life, including the existential questions about what gives their life meaning and purpose. They want to be able to talk about belief systems and about sexuality.

With empowerment comes responsibility. In the positive medicine model, patients become the experts in their own health, with support from their doctors. Empowerment comes with a sense of control and agency, a belief that you can take control of your circumstances. But there's no going back from that position. You can't blame the doctor if you don't do the things that you and your doctor have worked out will help you move forward with your life. In the person–doctor partnership, the requirement to own the end result rests with the patient.

Working through life's opportunities opens up choices. It may be that you reach a realization that things need to change in your life to move forward and experience life to the full. These can be difficult choices, with the rewards on the other side, but they are 'the road less travelled'. Many people settle for where they're at and don't make the tough calls. That's OK, particularly if it's a conscious choice. If you choose not to make tough calls, the most important thing is that you take control of the things that are within your power to control and enjoy life anyway.

One caution. There is a strong evidence base which demonstrates that taking control of one's life and applying the habits of positive health improves health, happiness, and length of life, and decreases illness and disease. However, that is a statistical finding that holds true for groups of people. I'm not proposing this model as a panacea, but I am saying it goes beyond what currently exists. The current medical model is losing the battle against illness and disease. What if the positive medicine process doesn't actually reduce your personal markers of disease (for instance, if it doesn't return the blood sugar of a type 2 diabetic to normal), but nonetheless the end result is understanding your own health better? What if the result is that you have more control of your life and a clearer sense of its purpose and meaning? What if the end result is that you feel happier?

Is that not a better outcome than the current deficit model of disease care, where the goal is to avoid a negative outcome?

Because this is a positive health model for health enhancement rather than a disease management model, it means that it applies to you whether you're fit and healthy and want to stay so (primary prevention), stressed and in a state of dis-ease with illness or disease waiting to happen (secondary prevention), or have already developed a condition or conditions (tertiary prevention). At any of these tiers, you are likely to benefit and be able to take control of your life and health.

What does this mean for doctors?

The RCGP in the UK is clear what general practice in the UK in 2030 needs to look and feel like, having undertaken extensive consultation. It will need new models of practice: 'Our vision is that by 2030, general practice will have the skills and resources it needs to meet the healthcare needs of the population by preventing more illness, diagnosing and treating disease and empowering patients to live healthy, fulfilling lives.'[13] The College describes more holistic, patient-centred models of care, focused more on prevention, adopting a partnership approach so that GPs can have more fulfilling relationships with their patients.

The RCGP foresees a team approach, with doctors providing just part of the picture, and incorporating other skills into the team, including helping people address the social determinants of health. There will be more flexibility and more use of technology, such as remote consultations (by phone or videoconference). As I work through their 2030 wish list, all the angles are covered by positive medicine. It ticks all the boxes. A model of practice such as positive medicine is the future of general practice in the UK by 2030, by my analysis.

This person–doctor partnership achieves a number of benefits for doctors as well as patients: because of the partnership approach, there is far more involvement from the patient in making management choices. This means more likelihood of therapeutic success and less inappropriate prescribing and risk of side effects. Greater levels of explanation and informed consent means lower utilization of treatment modalities lacking evidence, lower levels of dissatisfaction, and fewer patient complaints. It's safer for both patients and doctors.

My experience is of the privilege of spending time with people, hearing their stories, their hopes, and their fears. The fact that I can contribute and make a difference brings a huge degree of satisfaction. At our last session, my client Glyn said to me, 'I really look forward to our meetings. It feels as though I'm the focus of everything we're doing. It feels like a partnership.'

Again, I need to be clear that I don't see this model being for all doctors. I see it being ideal for GPs and some specialist doctors, such as occupational physicians, rehabilitation physicians, palliative care physicians (who practise to similar models in any case), and paediatricians. An obstetrician has just expressed interest in hearing more. I expect that some doctors will reject the approach as being too far removed from their training and their understanding of health and disease. My job is not to persuade them. Rather, I want to empower the doctors who tell me they are already aware of the need for more holistic and patient-centred models and want to practise to those models.

Where do the medical colleges fit in?

It is clear that the RCGP in the UK is taking a leadership role and seeking to positively influence the health of the population of the UK by new models of general practice. But 2030 is still a long way off. I suspect that the future vision it paints is so far off because of the inertia of the system, and the big change of emphasis required to move away from disease care to healthcare. I'm sure that the RCGP is already advocating for change at a system level. But it needs the strength of patient views and public opinion behind it in order to influence the political will to expedite change.

Here in New Zealand and Australia, the medical colleges have been under attack and accused of being simply a professional guild, established purely for the purpose of supporting their members; that the colleges are self-serving and not fit for purpose in the modern world of healthcare. Professor Des Gorman put forward this notion in the journal of the RACP.[14]

I see this challenge in the same light as that of Ivan Illich, and consider Professor Gorman to be a positive disruptor. He accuses the medical colleges of not responding to health system failings, of not reducing medical error, and asks the question:

Is the future college role to be constrained to professional and technical evaluation of doctor competence and up-skilling? Can the medical guilds become effective socially beyond intrinsic guild-need and play a role in preventing and mitigating, and in responding to health system failures?[15]

As an active and proud member of the RACP, my answer to Professor Gorman is a resounding 'Yes! I believe we can.'

As well as training and evaluating specialist physicians, the RACP is active in advocating for positive healthcare system change. Its EVOLVE project provides leadership in identifying the myriad of medical treatments and interventions with no proven value, and instead proven harm, and advocates for their use by doctors to be stopped. The Aotearoa New Zealand Committee of the RACP has been active in promoting action on healthy housing, good work, and family wellbeing. *Employment, Poverty and Health*, the statement of principles on the role of doctors to influence the social determinants of health, sets out the ways that doctors can move beyond traditional roles to have societal influence. And my own faculty has led the charge in developing the *Consensus Statement on the Health Benefits of Work*. The progression of the College's annual conference, Congress, shows how progressive its thinking is around health and practice. The RACP is active in health advocacy in its most holistic sense.

The medical colleges can be voices of advocacy for societal change and, in particular, addressing the challenges put to us by Ivan Illich. Illich saw patient pressure as the solution. That didn't work effectively against the system. The answer to iatrogenesis lies not with patients, but with doctors. Not just individual doctors, but the medical colleges. I personally challenge every board member of every medical college to read *Medical Nemesis* and, rather than reacting defensively, to critically appraise the case Illich puts forward for patient empowerment and new models of medical practice which reduce patient harm and increase people's ability to face life's challenges. If the argument was strong in the 1970s, I see it now as incontrovertible.

How is your college preparing to avoid impending nemesis?

Other key players

An underlying flaw in the system is the historical training of doctors. To achieve the future state, our medical students and junior doctors must able to practise the new principles and models of medical practice they are being taught. It follows that the universities and medical schools need to be influencing medical education, by communicating with the medical colleges which provide continuing professional development to doctors. I have been surprised talking to my own son and other medical students and junior doctors by just how different their training has been to my own, and the different concepts they are being taught. Yet these concepts are foreign to many senior doctors. This is a state of affairs which must not be allowed to continue.

The hospital system and those who design healthcare systems will be pricking their ears up. The potential for positive medicine as disruptive innovation leading to more effective, safer, and cheaper healthcare should be viewed as an opportunity for complete system redesign and revolutionary advances in healthcare, not the evolutionary improvement in disease care which is so obviously failing us. The opportunity for revolutionary change extends to hospital and local systems too, where innovative approaches can be taken.

Nurses and allied health professionals see the principles I espouse as obvious, because they reflect their own training. They completely understand the flaws of the medical model. That means there is an important role for the professional bodies of these non-doctor healthcare professionals to influence change and challenge the reductionist status quo of the medical model.

Others with a vested interest in getting this right include insurers, workers' or injury compensation bodies, lawyers, and employers. I see all these players as potentially adding to the flaws of the system. (In the thousands of cases where patients have been let down by the system, all of them have at times been contributory.) But being part of the problem always opens up the possibility of being part of the solution. I am seeing many large employers making great advances in looking after the health and wellbeing of their workers. I am seeing insurance companies taking a far more positive and health-promoting approach to insurance policies and claims management.

Ultimately, though, the solution does rest with the people, and specifically the representatives of the people. That power rests with government. As hard as it sometimes is to realize it, governments exist to deliver the will of the people and what is best for our communities and societies. That includes the departments and ministries of health, their chief scientists and chief medical advisors, and the civil servants who advise ministers and run government services. It is the political will which will ultimately decide the funding for new healthcare systems.

As patients, we *do* have a say, by making it clear to our politicians that we want positive change.

My response to Ivan Illich

Dear Ivan Illich,

In belated response to your 1974 warning of *Medical Nemesis*, I would like to apologize that we perceived your message as a threat, rather than the opportunity for change you intended.

As I write, 47 years later, patients are still asking for the empowerment and control over their lives and health that you warned was being taken from them by the medical system. You saw the root of the problem as being doctors. Iatrogenesis—it begins with the healer.

Ultimately, as you saw, the solution does rest with patients and their ability to influence political will and change systems. But there is a more elegant and powerful agent of change, and that is to go to the root of the problem, namely, doctors.

I propose that doctors provide the thought leadership for the revolutionary change to positive medicine in order to deliver the positive health that people are asking for. For doctors to go beyond the medical model to a holistic empowerment model means that the meaning of iatrogenesis can also be extended to reflect the shift in role—to positive iatrogenesis. Once again, it begins with the healer.

But here's the final twist. As we once again see doctors as the healers that society needs them to be, we also realize that we are all healers. Our body is the ultimate healer. Working together, the partnership creates the circumstances of ease to allow the body to heal. Since doctors are people too, and doctors are patients too, we all benefit. We are one.

Rehabilitation and Retention in the Workplace—The Interaction Between General Practitioners and Occupational Health Professionals: A Consensus Statement

Rehabilitation for work (vocational rehabilitation) is an extremely important issue. The growing emphasis placed on this by a range of stakeholders, including government, is welcome. This is an area that has been neglected in the UK for many years. For someone absent from work because of illness, or in work but with a disability, successful rehabilitation or adjustments in the workplace have a major impact on his or her health, well-being and position in society. For UK business and the country as a whole, there are enormous economic implications.

General practitioners (GPs) play a crucial role in this because they see many patients with chronic illness and disability, they co-ordinate and provide effective clinical management and they provide sick notes which trigger or continue periods of absence from work. Some GPs are not aware how influential their role is, or the beneficial effect that work can have on their patients' health. The GP's role may be compromised by time constraints, a lack of knowledge of the workplace and occupational health (OH) issues, and by apparent conflicts with their advocacy role, confidentiality and the doctor–patient relationship. Furthermore, there is no recognized structure within the UK National Health Service (NHS) for them to refer for OH advice.

For OH professionals (physicians and nurses), a core part of their role is assessment of functional ability against the requirements of the job and the workplace in order to provide advice to individuals and employers. Though they are retained by the employer, they are bound by a strict ethical code which puts the patient/employee's interests at the heart of their work. Their presence in the workplace is limited; however, where it exists there are examples of excellence in rehabilitation practice, but also of situations where influence and practice are lacking.

The ideal role in implementing the rehabilitation policy framework (which they should have played a part in establishing) is one of case manager; leading rehabilitation by assessment and liaison between individuals, GPs and other health care providers, managers, human resources and unions to advise on the measures required to remove the barriers to a successful return to work or retention in the workplace (including influences outside the medical model). There may be a training requirement to achieve this and other health professionals may also want to take on this role.

Communication between GPs and OH professionals is often very poor. Where it exists, there are examples of very good interaction, but in many cases it is non-existent. At its worst, it is adversarial, with suspicions of conflicting interests. This represents a significant barrier to rehabilitation, to the disadvantage of all concerned.

Overcoming this barrier will involve changes of attitude, culture and systems. This will require mutual education of GPs and OH professionals: looking at examples of best practice to increase understanding of what can be achieved in the workplace and the constraints of the 7 or 10 min appointment. The goal is a process by which GPs and OH professionals have a team approach to rehabilitation, with OH professionals acting as a source of advice or referral and liaising with the workplace as case manager.

We should aim for the situation where anyone off work for a sustained period is supported by a clear rehabilitation strategy, which they have been involved in developing. There will, however, be cases of serious illness where this is clearly inappropriate. This will require meaningful, two-way communication, including informal and face-to-face meetings where appropriate.

The many GPs who also work as occupational physicians or in medical education may be able to facilitate these changes. So, too, could the involvement of OH-trained practice nurses and initiatives such as OH projects which provide a bridge between the surgery and the workplace, along the lines of the Sheffield Occupational Health Advisory Service model in Sheffield.

Further parts of the process will include involvement of physiotherapists, occupational therapists, osteopaths, chiropractors and allied professionals with an influence on rehabilitation and closer liaison with Disability Services, Jobcentre Plus and other facilitators. The Disability Assessment doctors (who review cases for social security claims), many of whom are GPs, will also have much to offer this liaison and be able to influence their peers. Initiatives such as Securing Health Together and the Job Retention and Rehabilitation Pilots must receive the profile and funding they require for the ultimate development of greater rehabilitation resources nationally.

Rehabilitation is an issue with many stakeholders, each of whom must take ownership of their own role and continue to exert influence to improve the many areas that are currently lacking. A concerted team approach can bring about great benefits to individuals and society, some of which can be achieved with little financial outlay. This is the collective view of 25 key informants and stakeholders:

Carol Bannister, Royal College of Nursing Adviser in Occupational Health

Jamie Bell, Senior Policy Adviser, CBI

David Beswick, Medical Director, SchlumbergerSema Medical Services (Disability Assessment doctors)

John Challenor, President of the Society of Occupational Medicine

Ruth Chambers, Professor of Primary Care Development, Staffordshire University

Jim Ford, Medical Director, Job Retention and Rehabilitation Pilots, Department for Work and Pensions

Simon Fradd, Chairman, Doctor Patient Partnership and Joint Deputy Chair, General Practitioners Committee

Andrew Frank, President, British Society of Rehabilitation Medicine

Bill Gunnyeon, President, The Faculty of Occupational Medicine

Elizabeth Gyngell, Head of Health Strategy, Management and Research, Health & Safety Executive and Lead for Securing Health Together

David Haslam, Visiting Professor of Primary Health Care and Chairman of Council, Royal College of General Practitioners

Sharon Horan, Chair of the RCN Society of Occupational Health Nursing

Elizabeth Hughes, President, The Association of Occupational Health Nurse Practitioners (UK)

Paul Keen, Head of Disability Services and Financial Support Division, Jobcentre Plus

Ewan Macdonald, Chairman, Support Programme Action Group (PAG), Securing Health Together

Joe Neary, Chair of the Clinical Network, Royal College of General Practitioners

Simon Pickvance, Senior Occupational Health Adviser, Sheffield Occupational Health Advisory Service

David Pink, Chief Executive, Long Term Medical Conditions Alliance

David Powell, Assistant Manager Liability Insurance, Association of British Insurers (ABI)

Susan Robson, Chairman of the BMA Occupational Health Committee

Philip Sawney, Principle Medical Adviser, Corporate Medical Group, Department for Work and Pensions

Susan Scott-Parker, Chief Executive, Employers Forum on Disability

Diane Sinclair, Lead Adviser on Public Policy, Chartered Institute of Personnel and Development

Andy Slovak, Chief Medical Officer, BNFL

Owen Tudor, TUC Senior Policy Officer (Prevention, Rehabilitation and Compensation)

Consensus Statement on the Health Benefits of Good Work

At the heart of this consensus statement on the health benefits of good work is a shared commitment to improve the health and wellbeing of individuals, families and communities.

Good work is engaging, fair, respectful and balances job demands, autonomy and job security. Good work accepts the importance of culture and traditional beliefs. It is characterised by safe and healthy work practices and it strikes a balance between the interests of individuals, employers and society. It requires effective change management, clear and realistic performance indicators, matches the work to the individual and uses transparent productivity metrics.

Realising the health benefits of good work for all Australians and New Zealanders requires a transformation in both thought and in practice. It necessitates cooperation between a broad range of participants including workers, governments, employers, unions, insurers, legal practitioners, advocacy groups and healthcare professions.

Pledge

We, the undersigned, commit to collaboration, which encourages and enables Australians and New Zealanders to access the health benefits of good work. We acknowledge the following fundamental principles about the relationships between health and good work:

- The provision of good work is a key determinant of the health and wellbeing of employees, their families and broader society.
- Long term work absence, work disability and unemployment may have a negative impact on health and wellbeing.
- All workplaces should strive to be both healthy and safe.
- Providing access to good work is an effective means of reducing poverty and social exclusion.
- With active assistance, many of those who have the potential to work, but are not currently working, can be enabled to access the benefits of good work.
- Safe and healthy work practices, understanding and accommodating cultural and social beliefs, a healthy workplace culture, effective and equitable injury management programs and positive relationships within workplaces are key determinants of individual health, wellbeing, engagement and productivity.
- Good outcomes are more likely when individuals understand and are supported to access the benefits of good work, especially when entering the workforce for the first time, seeking re-employment or recovering at work following a period of injury or illness.

Governments, employers, workers, unions, insurers, legal practitioners, advocacy groups and healthcare professions all have a role in promoting the health benefits of good work.

Through actions appropriate to our various areas of responsibility or activity, we agree to:

- Promote an understanding of good work and an awareness of the health benefits of good work;
- Support and encourage those attempting to access the health benefits of good work;
- Encourage all participants to support workplace health; and
- Advocate for continuous improvement in public policy around work and health, consistent with the principles articulated above.

Australasian Faculty of Occupational and Environmental Medicine
Royal Australasian College of Physicians

Notes

Chapter 1

1. McKinstry, Brian. 'Paternalism and the doctor-patient relationship in general practice'. *The British Journal of General Practice*, 1992, 42(361): 340–342.
2. Neuberger, Julia. 'Let's do away with "patients"'. *BMJ*, 1999, 318(7200): 1756–1758.
3. McKinstry, 'Paternalism and the doctor-patient relationship in general practice'.
4. Au, Michelle. 'The radical notion that doctors are people too'. *Psychology Today*, 30 May 2011. https://www.psychologytoday.com/us/blog/wont-hurt-bit/201105/the-radical-notion-doctors-are-people-too.
5. European Patients' Forum. 'EPF Background Brief: Patient Empowerment', 15 May 2015. https://www.eu-patient.eu/globalassets/campaign-patient-empowerment/briefing_paperpatient-empowerment_final_external.pdf.
6. Ibid.

Chapter 2

1. Gration, John. 'Effective occupational health—difficulties of delivery'. *Occupational Medicine*, 1995, 45(2): 61–62.
2. Beaumont, David. 'The interaction between general practitioners and occupational health professionals in relation to return to work: a Delphi study'. *Occupational Medicine*, 2003, 53(4): 249–253.
3. Beaumont, David. 'Rehabilitation and retention in the workplace – the interaction between general practitioners and occupational health professionals'. *Occupational Medicine*, 2003, 53(4): 254–255.
4. Beach, Jeremy and David Watt. 'General practitioners and occupational health professionals'. *BMJ*, 2003, 327(7410): 302–303.
5. Cohen, Debbie, Naomi Marfell, Katie Webb, Mike Robling, and Mansel Aylward. 'Managing long-term worklessness in primary care: a focus group study'. *Occupational Medicine*, 2010, 60(2): 121–126.
6. https://www.racp.edu.au/docs/default-source/advocacy-library/realising-the-health-benefits-of-work.pdf (accessed 16 April 2020).
7. https://assets.publishing.service.gov.uk/government/uploads/system/uploads/attachment_data/file/209782/hwwb-working-for-a-healthier-tomorrow.pdf (accessed 14 April 2020).
8. https://assets.publishing.service.gov.uk/government/uploads/system/uploads/attachment_data/file/181060/health-at-work.pdf (accessed 14 April 2020).
9. Dr Kristin Good, personal correspondence.

Chapter 3

1. See https://www.rcgp.org.uk/-/media/Files/News/2019/RCGP-fit-for-the-future-report-may-2019.ashx?la=en (accessed 17 April 2020).

2. Illich, Ivan. *Limits to Medicine: Medical Nemesis: The Expropriation of Health*, 1975, p. 15. Also called *Limits to Medicine*.

3. Ibid., p. 3.

4. Ibid., p. 3.

5. Ibid., p. 271.

6. The data is available from NIDA, one of the National Institutes of Health, at https://www.drugabuse.gov/related-topics/trends-statistics/overdose-death-rates.

7. Illich, *Limits to Medicine*, p. 274.

8. Ibid., pp. 274–275.

9. Powles, John. 'On the limitations of modern medicine'. *Science, Medicine, and Man*, 1973, 1(1): 1–30.

10. Ibid., p. 25.

11. Engel, George. 'The need for a new medical model: a challenge for biomedicine'. *Science*, 1977, 196(4286): 129–136.

12. Ibid., p. 129.

13. Cohen Debbie, Naomi Marfell, Katie Webb, Mike Robling, and Mansel Aylward. 'Managing long-term worklessness in primary care: a focus group study'. *Occupational Medicine*, 2010, 60(2): 121–126.

14. Engel, 'The need for a new medical model', p. 129.

15. Balint, Michael. *The Doctor, His Patient and the Illness*, 2nd ed. New York: International Universities Press, 1972.

16. Guthrie, Else. 'Medically unexplained symptoms in primary care'. *Journal of Clinical Psychology*, 1998; 14: 432–440.

17. Reid, Steven, Simon Wessely, Tim Crayford, and Matthew Hotopf. 'Medically unexplained symptoms in frequent attenders of secondary health care: retrospective cohort study'. *BMJ*, 2001, 322(7289): 767.

Chapter 4

1. https://www.who.int/about/who-we-are/constitution.

2. Machteld Huber and colleagues proposed changing the emphasis towards the ability to adapt and self-manage in the face of social, physical, and emotional challenges. 'How should we define health?' Available from: https://www.researchgate.net/publication/51523299_How_should_we_define_health (accessed 18 April 2020).

3. Huber, M., M. van Vliet, M. Giezenberg, B. Winkens, Y. Heerkens, P.C. Dagnelie, and J.A. Knottnerus. 'Towards a patient-centred operationalisation of the new dynamic concept of health: a mixed-methods study'. *BMJ Open*, 2016, 5: e010091.

4. Ibid. 'We propose the concept of "positive health" ... elaborated from "health as the ability to adapt and self manage in the face of social, physical, and emotional challenges".'

5. Maslow, Abraham. 'A theory of human motivation'. *Psychological Review*, 1943, 50(4): 370–396.

6. Seligman, Martin. 'The new era of positive psychology'. TED talk; https://www.ted.com/talks/martin_seligman_the_new_era_of_positive_psychology?language=en.

7. Seligman, Martin. *Authentic Happiness: Using the New Positive Psychology to Realize your Potential for Lasting Fulfilment*. New York: Free Press, 2002.

8. Seligman, Martin. *Flourish: A Visionary New Understanding of Happiness and Wellbeing*. New York: Free Press, 2011.

9. See https://en.wikipedia.org/wiki/Maslow%27s_hierarchy_of_needs.

10. Maslow, Abraham H. *Motivation and Personality*, 3rd ed. New York: Harper & Row, 1987, p. 154.

Chapter 5

1. Lucy later added, after reading the manuscript of this book: 'Upon reflection, I have the awareness and the confidence to express myself because I'm fortunate: although some medical practitioners see me as my disability, my key medical contact/specialist (my neurosurgeon), along with my parents, treated me particularly through my early years in a very proactive and encouraging way. This has allowed me to see how things can be done and how things can be further improved; along with how some aspects of people's approach to disability is seriously lacking.'

2. https://www.who.int/topics/disabilities/en/.

3. https://www.iasp-pain.org/Education/Content.aspx?ItemNumber=1698.

4. The IASP defines central sensitization like this: 'Increased responsiveness of nociceptive neurons in the central nervous system to their normal or subthreshold afferent input.'

5. *Cole's Medical Practice in New Zealand*, 12 ed., 2013, p.39.

6. https://icd.who.int/browse11/l-m/en#/http://id.who.int/icd/entity/794195577.

Chapter 6

1. Antonovsky, Aaron. *Health, Stress, and Coping*. San Francisco, CA: Jossey-Bass, 1979.

2. Felitti, Vincent J., Robert F. Anda, Dale Nordenberg, David F. Williamson, Alison M. Spitz, Valerie Edwards, Mary P. Koss, et al. 'Relationship of childhood abuse and household dysfunction to many of the leading causes of death in adults'. *American Journal of Preventive Medicine*, 1998, 14(4): 245–258.

3. There is a summary of the interview with Professor Sheldon Cohen on the website of Carnegie Mellon University: https://www.cmu.edu/homepage/health/2012/spring/stress-on-disease.shtml.

4. You can watch Professor Sir Mason Durie's oration at: https://www.youtube.com/watch?v=2PcjRzNeKF4.

5. Durie, Mason. 'A Māori perspective of health'. *Social Science and Medicine*, 1985, 20(5): 483–486.

6. Chambers, Charlotte. 'Burnout in New Zealand's senior medical profession'. *The Specialist*, 2016, 108: 3. Available at: https://www.asms.org.nz/wp-content/uploads/2016/10/11210-The-Specialist-Issue-108-WEB.pdf.

7. https://www.wma.net/policies-post/wma-declaration-of-geneva/.

Chapter 7

1. https://www.racp.edu.au/advocacy/policy-and-advocacy-priorities/employment-poverty-and-health.
2. Van Roode, Thea, Nigel Dickson, Peter Herbison, and Charlotte Paul. 'Child sexual abuse and persistence of risky sexual behaviours and negative sexual outcomes over adulthood'. *Child Abuse and Neglect*, 2009, 33(33): 161–172.
3. Sacks, Vanessa and David Murphey. 'The prevalence of adverse childhood experiences, nationally, by state, and by race or ethnicity'. 2018. Available from Center for Victim Research Repository: https://www.childtrends.org/publications/prevalence-adverse-childhood-experiences-nationally-state-race-ethnicity http://hdl.handle.net/20.500.11990/1142.
4. Brady, David M. *The Fibro Fix: Get to the Root of your Fibromyalgia*. Emmaus, PA: Rodale Press, 2016, p. 14.
5. https://www.fibrofix.com.
6. See, for instance, https://www.health.harvard.edu/mental-health/the-power-of-the-placebo-effect or https://www.medicalnewstoday.com/articles/306437 for an overview of the evidence.
7. https://www.nhs.uk/news/medical-practice/survey-finds-97-of-gps-prescribe-placebos/.
8. For instance, a study by the Mayo Clinic in the US of patients seeking second opinions found that more than 20 per cent had been misdiagnosed, while 66 per cent required some changes to their diagnoses. See Van Such, Monica, Robert Lohr, Thomas Beckman, and James M. Naessens. 'Extent of diagnostic agreement among medical referrals'. *Journal of Evaluation in Clinical Practice*, 2017, 23(4): 870–874.
9. Durie, Mason. 'A Māori perspective of health'. *Social Science and Medicine*, 1985, 20(5): 483–486.
10. Best, Megan, et al. 'Why do we find it so hard to discuss spirituality? A qualitative exploration of attitudinal barriers'. *Journal of Clinical Medicine*, 2016, 5(9): 77.
11. Ibid.
12. Durie, 'A Māori perspective of health'. See also https://www.health.govt.nz/our-work/populations/maori-health/maori-health-models/maori-health-models-te-whare-tapa-wha.
13. Best et al., 'Why do we find it so hard to discuss spirituality?'.
14. Ibid.
15. Haboubi, N.H.J. and N. Lincoln. 'Views of health professionals on discussing sexual issues with patients'. *Disability and Rehabilitation*, 2003, 25(6): 291–296.

Chapter 8

1. Ellen Langer's research is described at: https://www.nytimes.com/2014/10/26/magazine/what-if-age-is-nothing-but-a-mind-set.html.
2. Blackburn, Elizabeth. *The Telomere Effect*. New York: Grand Central Publishing, 2017, p. 6.
3. Ibid.

4. Sinclair, David. *Lifespan: Why We Age—and Why We Don't Have To*. New York: Atria Books, 2019.
5. See https://thefast800.com/?gclid=EAIaIQobChMIoaOZxM-86QIVFKmWCh0 cEwDnEAAYAiAAEgLJZ_D_BwE.
6. See https://whatthefatbook.com/author/grant/.

Chapter 9

1. Durie, Mason. 'A Māori perspective of health'. *Social Science and Medicine*, 1985, 20(5): 483–486.
2. Dalai Lama. https://www.dalailama.com/messages/compassion-and-human-values/ compassion.
3. Government Inquiry into Mental Health and Addiction. *He Ara Oranga: Report of the Government Inquiry into Mental Health and Addiction*. November 2018. Available at: https://mentalhealth.inquiry.govt.nz/inquiry-report/he-ara-oranga/.
4. Ibid., p. 9.
5. See the Budget summary at: https://treasury.govt.nz/publications/wellbeing-budget/ wellbeing-budget-2019-html.
6. The phrase is attributed to a poem by the sixteenth-century Spanish mystic, St John of the Cross, known as 'La noche oscura del alma'. You may know it via T.S. Eliot (Four Quartets) or even Douglas Adams.
7. See https://www.racp.edu.au/docs/default-source/advocacy-library/realising-the-health-benefits-of-work.pdf.

Chapter 10

1. Larkin, Philip. 'This be the verse'. *High Windows*. London: Faber and Faber, 1974.
2. Katie, Byron—see https://thework.com.
3. https://www.ted.com/talks/brene_brown_the_power_of_vulnerability.
4. Brown, Brené. *The Gifts of Imperfection*. Center City, MN: Hazelden, 2010, p. 1.

Chapter 11

1. Cobb, Mark R., Christina M. Puchalski, and Bruce Rumbold. *Oxford Textbook of Spirituality in Healthcare*. Oxford: Oxford University Press, 2012.
2. van den Bosch, Matilda and William Bird (eds.). *Oxford Textbook of Nature and Public Health*. Oxford: Oxford University Press, 2018.
3. 'Thwarting, actual or imminent, of these basic needs provides a psychological threat that leads to psychopathy.' Maslow, Abraham H. 'A theory of human motivation'. *Psychological Review*, 1943, 50(4): 370–396.
4. Ibid., p. 370.
5. Peck, M. Scott. *The Road Less Travelled*. New York: Simon & Schuster, 1978.

Epilogue

1. Illich, Ivan. *Limits to Medicine: Medical Nemesis*. London: Calder & Boyars, 1974.
2. Iatrogenesis, from the Greek iatros (doctor), meaning 'inadvertent harm caused by doctors'. Illich defined three levels: firstly, clinical iatrogenesis, which includes the harm done directly by doctors, including ineffective, unsafe, and erroneous treatments; secondly, social iatrogenesis, the medicalization of normal life events such as ageing; and thirdly, cultural iatrogenesis, the destruction of traditional ways of dealing with death, suffering, and sickness.
3. Illich, Ivan. *Limits to Medicine: Medical Nemesis*, 2nd ed. London: Calder & Boyars, 1995, pp. v–vi.
4. Illich, Ivan. *Deschooling Society*. London: Marion Boyars, 1971.
5. https://www.ted.com/talks/sir_ken_robinson_do_schools_kill_creativity?language=en.
6. https://www.envano.com/learn/personas/positive-disruptor/#:~:text=%5Bpoz%2Di%2Dtiv%20dis,our%20day%2Dto%2Dday.
7. Marshall Marinker's obituary: https://www.thelancet.com/journals/lancet/article/PIIS0140-6736(19)31729-5/fulltext.
8. https://jme.bmj.com/content/medethics/1/2/81.full.pdf.
9. Marshall Marinker's obituary, https://www.thelancet.com/journals/lancet/article/PIIS0140-6736(19)31729-5/fulltext.
10. https://jme.bmj.com/content/medethics/1/2/81.full.pdf.
11. Illich, Ivan. 'Medical nemesis'. *The Lancet*, 1974, 303(7863): 918–921.
12. Illich, Ivan. *Limits to Medicine: Medical Nemesis*, 2nd ed. London: Calder & Boyars, 1995, p. 274.
13. https://www.rcgp.org.uk/-/media/Files/News/2019/RCGP-fit-for-the-future-report-may-2019.ashx?la=en.
14. Gorman, Des. 'Medical colleges: whose purpose, if any, do they serve?' *Internal Medicine Journal*, 2017, 47(3): 245–247.
15. Ibid.

Index

For the benefit of digital users, indexed terms that span two pages (e.g., 52–53) may, on occasion, appear on only one of those pages.

Notes

vs. indicates a comparis on. Figures are indicated by *f* following the page number